From the H
Your Mental Health Questi

PROFESSOR PATRICIA CASEY

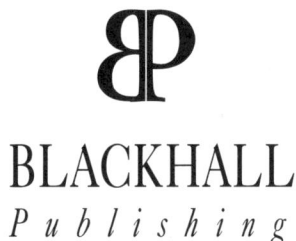

BLACKHALL
Publishing

This book was typeset by Gough Typesetting for
Blackhall Publishing
27 Carysfort Avenue
Blackrock
Co. Dublin
Ireland

e-mail: info@blackhallpublishing.com
www.blackhallpublishing.com

© Patricia Casey, 2004

ISBN: 1 842180 79 7

A catalogue record for this book is available from the British Library.

All rights reserved. No part of this publication may be reproduced, stored in a retrieval system or transmitted in any form or by any means, electronic, mechanical, photocopying, recording or otherwise, without the prior, written permission of the publisher.

This book is sold subject to the condition that it shall not, by way of trade or otherwise, be lent, resold, hired out, or otherwise circulated without the publisher's prior consent in any form of binding or cover other than that in which it is published and without a similar condition including this condition being imposed on the subsequent purchaser.

Printed in Ireland by
ColourBooks Ltd

*To John, James and Gavan
for your patience and love*

Contents

Acknowledgements ix

Introduction xi

Alternative Therapies 1

Anxiety Disorders 11

Bereavement 41

Dementia 57

Depression and Manic-Depression 67

Eating Disorders 101

Insomnia 107

Medico-Legal 115

Miscellaneous 135

Personality Disorders 153

Psychiatric Services 165

Psychological Therapies 177

Psychosexual Disorders 185

Schizophrenia 203

Somatoform Disorders 221

Stress 229

Substance Abuse 241

Suicide 265

Index 281

Acknowledgements

I have been privileged to have given lectures on various aspects of mental health in cities, towns and villages throughout this county and many people have written to me with specific queries. Their appetite and thirst for information, born out of concern for those with mental health problems, is striking and it is this that has led me to compile this volume.

I am grateful to everybody who has taken time to come out on cold, wet, winter nights to my talks, to all those who have read my weekly column and written to me and to the many courageous people who have spoken publicly about their own difficulties. Without you, this book would not have come about.

I am indebted to Gerry O'Regan, editor of the *Evening Herald*, and to Frank Coughlan, associate editor, and Dave Lawlor, features editor, who have given me a platform from which to address these issues in the column "From the Heart". I am grateful to Blackhall Publishing for having faith that this book would be of help to others and for their tremendous assistance throughout the production period.

Introduction

Mental health problems are common, distressing and disabling. Those who experience them are often stigmatised and regarded as different from others in a way that is distinct from those with other medical conditions. There is also a significant degree of misunderstanding about the causes of these disorders, about their treatment and about the health professionals who treat them.

Psychiatric disorders are unique in that their very existence is questioned by many, in spite of the emotional burden that they impose on the sufferer, their families and on society as a whole. Fear is one of the driving forces behind these negative attitudes, making them difficult to challenge and overcome.

There is a substantial body of research demonstrating that the best antidote to fear is knowledge. Those who have personal knowledge of or contact with mental health problems are the least likely to feel fearful or ashamed.

This book was compiled with the aim of challenging the negative stereotypes that are frequently applied to those who have mental health problems. Furthermore it is hoped that it will provide information to the public on a range of problems and disorders so that they will be in a better position to identify hidden difficulties and seek appropriate help.

At a time when the public is rightly demanding more information on the range of issues that confront us in our daily lives, a book such as this will, hopefully, fill a lacuna in an area that is seldom talked about except in hushed tones.

Mental health problems differ in their impact – sometimes there is emotional pain, other times there is impaired functioning and sometimes there may be unawareness that such a problem exists in spite of obvious incapacity. Since the effects are complex we hope this book will provide some answers for those with mental health problems and for their families. However, this book should not substitute professional help. We would like to emphasise that the *publisher, author and their colleagues quoted in this book disclaim any liability* for any pain, injury, unpleasantness, stress or other negative reactions or outcomes that may result from the use, proper or improper, of the information, suggestions or directives in this book. We do not guarantee that the information given herein is complete, nor should it be considered as a substitute for the reader's common sense or good judgement in seeking professional help. The information in this book must not be construed or interpreted to infringe on the rights of others or to violate the laws of the land.

Alternative Therapies

Alternative therapies carry no risks.

Common myth

Alternative Therapies

I am a healthcare worker, attached to a general practice. Patients frequently complain that they are being given antidepressants and tranquillizers by their doctors and that they will not even consider alternative remedies. Surely if enough people want and use a particular medicine and it appears to be safe, that should be enough to justify prescribing it.

Many people feel that they would prefer alternative medicines and these have achieved a lot of publicity in recent years. One of the requirements of doctors is that they are obliged to use the best treatments available for their patients and those that are licensed for use by the Irish Medicines Board. If a particular medicine is not licensed then there must be very good reasons for prescribing it instead of those that are licensed. The reason for this is that unlicensed medicines might have unacceptable side effects, they might interact with other drugs or alcohol or they might be no more effective than inert substances, known as placebos. There are also obvious medico-legal implications.

Licensing

The licensing of a drug requires proof that the drug has been through several stages in its testing. The first is the laboratory phase where it is tested on animals. Many drugs fail at this stage as serious side effects emerge. For those that pass this phase, the next stage involves healthy volunteers being administered the product to rule out the possibility of serious side effects in humans. Then it must be tested in controlled trials against placebos. This means clearly selecting the patient group in whom it is to be tested. So, for example, if an antidepressant is being developed, it is essential to define the symptoms that must be present and their severity. A placebo is used against which to compare it and although this surprises many, up to 30 per cent of patients respond to a placebo. In these trials neither patient nor doctor knows who is given active drug and who is given placebo. Needless to say, all of this information is given to the patient so that full consent can be given. The next phase involves comparing the new drug with those already in use for the same condition. It is only at that point, when a large enough sample of patients has received the drug in these controlled conditions, that a licence for its use will be issued.

Alternative Medicines

St John's Wort has been tested in a number of trials which suggest that it may be effective in the treatment of mild to moderate depression. However, there is reason for continuing caution, since the trials have flaws in them, among them the low dose of the comparison drugs that were used and the lack of trials comparing it with the most commonly used antidepressants. Furthermore, the studies are short – trials of most other antidepressants last for at least twelve weeks whereas studies of St John's Wort to date last no longer than a few weeks. Although it has not been shown to be unhelpful in treating severe depression it is possible that with better studies the present findings for its use at the milder end of the spectrum will be upheld and it can be prescribed more confidently.

Omega-3 oil is found in fish oils and again has not been tested in a sufficiently large number of trials as yet. However, a recent study comparing it against placebo did find it to be effective in those who had failed to respond to other antidepressants. However, as this was an isolated study, more are clearly needed before it could be licensed. Some studies also suggest that it is helpful in treating schizophrenia that has not fully responded to existing medication and it is tentatively recommended for use in combination with established medication.

Active Ingredients

Even natural products have active ingredients that act on the brain cells and nerve endings. It is these ingredients that bring about the improvement. For example, omega-3 oil has two active ingredients that act on the coating of the nerves whilst St John's Wort has at least ten different components. One of the problems is that there is no definite certainty as to which one is active in treating depression.

* * *

So it is not that doctors are being deliberately obstructive in depriving their patients of these natural remedies, but that conclusive information about their effectiveness and safety is lacking. In fact, one of the oldest drugs in psychiatry is lithium, a naturally occurring substance that is used to treat manic-depression and depression. It has been in use since 1967.

Useful Reading

Ernst, E., Pittler, M.H., Stevinson, C. et al. (2001) *The Desktop Guide to Complementary and Alternative Medicine*, Harcourt: London

Alternative Therapies

I am thirty and have been suffering with depression for several months. My doctor prescribed an antidepressant for me and I have no problem with this except that I am not getting any better. I wonder if St John's Wort would be better. I like the idea of taking a natural remedy to treat my condition. Also, as I hope to become pregnant in the next few months I thought this might be safer than the usual antidepressants. Can you advise me?

I am sorry that you are depressed and not getting better. Usually, recovery from depression is quite rapid, occurring over a few weeks. I can fully understand why you might be considering taking the "natural" route.

Effective

The active ingredient in St John's Wort is hypericum and several studies have indeed shown it to be effective in the treatment of mild to moderate depression, i.e. depression that is not so debilitating that time has to be taken off work or that extra help at home is needed. The symptoms you experience may also be a guide. If you have lost weight, have early morning wakening and feel worse at that time of day you may have a form of depression once known as melancholia that does not respond very well to hypericum. If you have suicidal thoughts, and I assume you do not as you are planning a family, then this treatment is not suitable. Since I do not have a lot of information on the effect this illness is having on your daily life I cannot say for certain but you may be suitable for this treatment.

Drug and Food Interactions

It is often assumed that natural remedies have no chemical effects. In fact St John's Wort is very like two groups of antidepressants. The first is the group to which "prozac" belongs, termed the SSRIs, and the second a much older group, the MAOIs, of which "nardil" is the best known.

If you do begin St John's Wort, there will have to be a gap of one to two weeks between stopping your present treatment and commencing the new one, depending on the treatment you are presently on. The reason for this is that St John's Wort interacts with a number of medications including the oral contraceptive, anti-clotting drugs, antidepressants and over-the-counter preparations such as nasal decongestants.

St John's Wort contains hypericum, which inhibits monoamine-oxidase, a chemical associated with depression, and this may potentially lead to serious interactions with food and drinks including alcohol, sour cream, aged or canned meats, liver, meat extracts, salami, sausage, cheese, smoked food such as smoked mackerel or salmon, herring, broad beans and possibly yoghurt. It is unclear from the data if dietary restrictions should be put in place as with some other antidepressants known as the monoamine-oxidase inhibitors (MAOIs).

Risks

There has not been a lot of research into St John's Wort so there is no information on its safety during pregnancy or if it is excreted in breast milk. As you are considering pregnancy, this is something to be considered. Although it can work within two weeks, the onset of action may take up to twelve weeks, which is slightly longer than with conventional antidepressants. The side effects include nausea, restlessness and anxiety. Occasionally, sensitivity to light can lead to an allergic rash. Overall, it compares favourably with other antidepressants in its profile of side effects.

Caution

St John's Wort is not prescribed much by doctors, as there is a dearth of research into its complications, safety and interactions with other drugs. As it is now no longer available across the counter, your doctor would have to prescribe it. The local medicine's boards do not regulate preparations bought abroad in health-food shops or through the Internet and so the purity of the preparation that you receive cannot be guaranteed. This may mean that the content of the important ingredient, hypericum, varies with the source.

* * *

Whatever treatment you opt for, I hope you get well soon and that your future plans will be realised.

Useful Websites

www.hypericum.acom

www.vh.org/adult/patient/psychiatry/medications/stjohn.html

My general practitioner tells me that I am suffering from depression and wants to prescribe antidepressants. However, I do not want to take medication and I wonder if hypnosis would be helpful. A friend of mine went to a hypnotherapist for smoking and she has done very well and another friend who has anxiety was also helped. Can you tell me something about hypnosis, as I have some fears about it?

I would advise you to consider carefully what your general practitioner has advised, as she knows you well and is in a very good position to recommend the best treatment for you. Your doctor cannot recommend a treatment that has not been scientifically shown to be effective for your illness, since that would be unethical. In addition, depression can be severe or long lasting if it is not treated appropriately.

Uses

Hypnotherapy is not widely used for psychiatric problems in this country and only a handful of psychiatrists practise it. It has been used with varying degrees of success to treat obesity and substance abuse disorders such as alcoholism. Its greatest use is now probably in the management of smoking and its discontinuation. Occasionally, it is used to induce anaesthesia and although major surgery has seldom been carried out using hypnosis in this country, a number of dentists do use it.

It has also been used to treat anxiety-related disorders such as generalised anxiety and phobias with some success, since it induces a state of relaxation that will allow the individual expose themselves to the feared situation. In relation to your specific query about depression, I am not aware of it having any major role in its treatment and certainly, there are no controlled studies that I am aware of to examine its effectiveness.

Hypnotic Induction

A session begins by "inducing" the hypnotic state. Various techniques may be used, such as the swinging watch, although this is rarely used now. More commonly the person is asked to glance upwards at their eyebrows and as the eyelids move to allow the eyes to close. Persons under hypnosis are in a trance state. In a light trance the person feels relaxed and tingling of the skin can be induced. A medium trance is associated with diminished pain while a deep trance is associated with anaesthesia and time distortion. Post-hypnotic suggestion, following from a deep trance state, refers to the instruction to perform a simple act or to experience a particular sensation after awakening.

For example, it may be used to give a bad taste to food thus helping in the treatment of obesity. There is still uncertainty as to whether a person can carry out acts during a hypnotic trance that are repugnant to their morals, although most hynotherapists will say that this is not possible.

Dangers

As with any intervention, even those that seem benign and drug free, there are dangers with hypnosis. Because the patient is in a state of dependence on the therapist, which is greater and certainly different from other therapeutic relationships, the possibility of a strong attachment between the therapist and patient must be borne in mind. Those who have difficulties with trust or who have problems giving up control are not good candidates for hypnosis, since negative feelings about the therapist can emerge. Those who suffer with psychotic illnesses such as manic-depression or schizophrenia are also vulnerable to recurrences after hypnosis.

Suggestibility

Especially when in a deep trance patients are malleable and suggestible and in this state memories that have been forgotten can be recalled. Freud used it to help patients recover memories that had been "repressed". However, there is some controversy as to whether these memories are recalled as they actually happened or whether they are changed or elaborated upon so as to distort them. In this state it is believed false memories can be suggested. Using hypnotherapy to reclaim lost memories may thus lead to the syndrome known as "false memory syndrome". Not only is this distressing for the patient but it can splinter families and create legal problems if this material is used in a court of law in this country.

* * *

I strongly recommend you speak again with your doctor and you should contact a reputable hypnotherapy organisation. There is no convincing evidence that hypnotherapy has a role in treating depression and you should remember that because a therapy works in one condition does not necessarily mean that it will be effective in others.

Useful Website

www.brooksidecenter.com

Useful Contact

Irish Institute of Counselling and Hypnotherapy
118 Stillorgan Road, Dublin 4, Tel. (01) 2600118

Anxiety Disorders

The only thing we have to fear is fear itself – nameless, unjustified terror which paralyses needed efforts to convert retreat into advance.

Franklyn D. Roosevelt,
Inaugural Address, 1933

I am thirty-two years old and for the past eighteen months I have been having trouble leaving my house. In fact, I am almost totally housebound. It began after I was chased by a vicious dog on my way home from work. Although I was not bitten and the owners got rid of the animal, I have been terrified ever since. I manage to go to work but my husband has to take me and collect me. In fact, I can't even do the weekly shopping unless he is with me and my children have to go to the local shops for me. My family are just wonderful as they do everything for me that involves going out. Strangely enough, I feel fine at home unless I know I have to go out. I feel totally helpless to fight this.

From your description I think you are probably suffering from agoraphobia, which means, literally, fear of the marketplace. This is relatively common and affects about 2 per cent of the population. So you are not alone. Although your main fear is of leaving your home, for many people there is also a fear of crowds, of telephone kiosks or of any enclosed space.

Good News

As has happened in your case, this condition sometimes begins following a frightening event and it has been known to begin even in the teenage years. If it is not treated it fluctuates, so that from time to time the sufferer will seem to improve only to have a recurrence.

The good news is that this is a treatable condition and since it has not begun until well into adulthood the prospect of you making a complete recovery is very high. The main form of treatment is termed behaviour therapy and your general practitioner will advise you on how best to access this. Treatment may take a few months and will not involve medication.

Self-Help

While you are waiting for treatment to begin there are some things you can do to help yourself. The Out and About Organisation is devoted to helping and treating those with agoraphobia and you should make contact with them. Also, your family, although they are very helpful, may unwittingly be making your phobia worse, as they are removing the motivation for you to begin trying to go out. This ironically is one of the drawbacks of having a very supportive family. You should ask them to encourage you to go out and even to accompany you from a distance rather than doing everything for you.

Graded Exposure

You could also help yourself by making a list of all the situations that you find difficult and then grading them in relation to the amount of anxiety they cause you. For example, you might find that going to your front door is easier than going to the bottom of the garden and this may be easier than walking on the footpath. This is termed a hierarchy. By tackling each feared situation on the list, beginning at the easiest, and practising it until you have mastered it without fear, you will gradually overcome your fears. Each step may take a day or even two but the crucial thing is to move to the next step only when you feel ready. Moving up the hierarchy in this manner is termed graded exposure. If you feel tense, especially before you begin the exposure, you should do relaxation exercises and this will make the process a little easier.

On no account must you try to overcome your greatest fear at the outset, as this will lead to panic attacks. When you have mastered each situation you must keep on practising it. If you feel unable to use this approach yourself then your therapist will work with you to achieve this, since this is the most common approach used by behaviour therapists to treat agoraphobia.

Rewards

It is important to reward yourself – a small treat every week will encourage you in your endeavours. Do not get downhearted if things appear to be moving too slowly as the whole process may take several months.

* * *

There is no magical cure or medication to overcome your agoraphobia. The sooner you seek professional help the better, since the longer the phobia is established the harder it is to overcome it. You have had your phobia for about eighteen months and that is a relatively short time. So good luck and look forward to being able to go out as you did before this problem began.

Useful Reading

Elaine Sheehan (1996) *Anxiety: Phobias and Panic Attacks*, Element Books: London

Useful Website

www.epub.org.br/cm/n05/doencas/fobias_i.htm

Useful Contact

Out and About Organisation
140 St Lawrence's Road, Clontarf, Dublin 11, Tel. (01) 8338252

I have been having problems at home recently and as a result I am having difficulty getting off to sleep. I am also much more tense than usual and cannot stop worrying about my problems. My family doctor has given me a prescription for tranquillizers but I am frightened to take them without some more information, as I was never keen on tablets anyway. Can you help please?

I am sorry that you are not feeling well at present. If you are not sleeping and therefore feeling tired all the time, coping even with minor problems can be difficult. Also, if you are constantly worrying you are probably not able to get enough "distance" between you and your difficulties to examine solutions. It is important to remember that you may need professional help from a therapist to deal with these issues and that tablets in themselves may not help in the long term. However, for the moment, it is probably a good idea to take the medication prescribed by your doctor. You should begin by reading the patient information leaflet that legally must accompany all medications.

Major and Minor Tranquillizers

Confusion often arises about the term "tranquillizer" since some of the treatments used in schizophrenia are termed major tranquillizers and include drugs such as chlorpromazine and haloperidol. Interestingly, these are not associated with dependence, although they have other side effects such as restless legs syndrome and stiffness.

The benzodiazepines, which you have been prescribed, are called minor tranquillizers and they work by attaching themselves to nerve endings in the brain known as benzodiazepine receptors. They are used in a wide variety of conditions other than anxiety, including epilepsy and restless leg syndrome (known as akathisia); they are also used as muscle relaxants and prior to surgery. There are three major types of these medications: short-, medium- and long-acting – depending on the length of time they remain in the body.

Preventing Dependence

One of the difficulties with minor tranquillizers, as distinct from antidepressants, is that they are associated with dependence. However, if you take them only when you need them rather than as a regular prescription then this is much less a possibility. You could also vary the dose once you know how you are reacting to them. The best way to prevent dependence is to take them for no longer than four to six weeks. In general, the short-acting benzodiazepines are the most likely to produce withdrawal reactions so the long acting ones are the safest in terms of ease of discontinuation. As I do not know which benzodiazepine you were prescribed I cannot tell you to which group it belongs but your patient information sheet, contained in the packet, will do so.

If your problems are continuing and you are unable to deal with them in spite of this treatment then you need to find additional ways of coping such as using relaxation exercises or talking to a professional about solutions.

Caution

In general, when taken on their own for a limited period benzodiazepines are very safe. However, if they are combined with alcohol or with other medications they can cause drowsiness and if taken in an overdose with these drugs they may also have serious consequences. Those working with machinery would also need to adjust the dose if drowsy, since safety may be a concern.

* * *

Overall, you do not need to have too many concerns if you take the medication only as you need it and for a limited period of time with no other medications.

Useful Reading

Ling, W., Smith, D.E. and Wesson, D. (1994) *Prescription Drug Abuse and Addiction: Answering your Questions*, Hazelden Publishing and Educational Services: USA

Useful Website

www.tranx.org.au/benzodiaz.html

I have recently started worrying about things. By nature I am laid-back but now I fret about everything. My husband says I need help as I have no real problems yet I am having trouble coping every day. My general practitioner has suggested tranquillizers but I am reluctant to take medication and I would rather manage without it. What do you suggest?

There are several points about worry that may be pertinent to you. Worry is a natural reaction to events and problems that arise. In fact, in some instances it would be abnormal not to worry. For example, if your children are causing problems or you have financial difficulties it is understandable that you would react by thinking about them and in doing this try to work out solutions. However, some people are "born worriers" and will over-react to everyday events or will look for problems when there are none.

Usually Laid-Back

You are lucky that you are not of an anxious disposition, as this is very difficult to treat. If the worrying does not seem to come from your personality or from any real problems in your life and there is no obvious explanation for it you may indeed be in need of professional help. This is especially so if it is affecting your life. Are you sleeping less than before? Are you getting forgetful? These are common symptoms in those who are worried and preoccupied. Sometimes panic attacks can occur in response to excessive worry. Do you feel tired even after a good night's sleep? What are your spirits like? Have you lost weight or needed time off work? Are you able to cope with the housework or do you need to get help with this also? These are some of the questions that are relevant to establishing the cause of these symptoms.

Causes

A number of conditions can cause excessive worrying when there isn't really a cause. An anxiety disorder called generalised anxiety can be responsible. This is a common condition and feeling tense and sleeping less are the main symptoms. Depressive illness can also cause excessive worrying, even when the depressed mood is not obvious. Feelings of tiredness, aches and pains, and poor concentration are among the symptoms to look out for. In addition, when depression is present the person often feels tearful for no reason and confidence drops. Finally, an overactive thyroid gland can also cause anxiety of the type you describe and a simple blood test can diagnose this condition. Sometimes people speak of stress as a cause of excessive worry but unless you have specific problems to be concerned about then this is not a cause of your present difficulties.

Medication

The necessity for medication depends on the diagnosis. For example, antidepressants are very helpful and not addictive if the cause is a depressive illness. If it is caused by thyroid problems, then this is a medical and not a psychiatric condition and responds to specific treatment to reduce the activity in the thyroid gland. Finally, if it is caused by an anxiety state then tranquillizers may be needed in the short term, but they have their own potential problems.

Alternatives

Relaxation exercises or yoga can assist in reducing your anxiety level. However, this depends on how severe your tension and anxiety is. Some people, try as they may, cannot settle sufficiently to get involved with the exercise regime. If this happens you might consider short-term medication to help your initial engagement with relaxation techniques. Exercise can also reduce tension, as can prayer and meditation. Try playing some restful music or listening to sounds of nature such as running streams – these are available commercially on CD now.

* * *

Ultimately, you must visit your doctor again and discuss the diagnosis and whether these non-drug-related options are possible. I hope that you feel well quickly and I am confident that with appropriate treatment, you will.

Useful Reading

Marks, Isaac (2002) *Living with Fear*, McGraw Hill: Maidenhead, England

Useful Website

www.google.com
(Key in "Royal College of Psychiatrists" and then "anxiety" – there is an excellent essay devoted to coping with anxiety)

I am a thirty-three-year-old mother of two lovely children. I often get very strange feelings and my doctor says he does not know what the cause is, as he has never come across this before. Every few weeks I get a feeling of detachment from everything around me. I know what is going on, I can see and hear, but it is as if I am "outside" myself and not really part of what is going on. I pinch myself to try to re-connect but I just have to wait for it to pass spontaneously. I am very worried about this.

I can understand how perplexing this must be for you, as you have no name for these episodes. It is a frightening condition, especially if it lasts for longer than a few moments and people often react like you do, with fears for their well-being.

Depersonalisation

What you describe is called "depersonalisation" and it is a relatively common phenomenon. It can occur when people are very tired or when they are hungry. Sometimes a hangover can cause it. It may also be associated with severe anxiety or occasionally depression. Also, those who are coming off tranquillizers, such as diazepam, can experience depersonalisation. Severe stress such that soldiers experience in combat may also cause it, as it serves as a type of short-term psychological protection. In a few, very rare instances, it can occur as a disorder in its own right. However, in most instances it is a perfectly normal occurrence and studies have shown that it can occur as an isolated phenomenon in up to 70 per cent of people.

Derealisation

Sometimes the condition can be confused with a phenomenon called *deja vu* – when the person feels that they have experienced the present moment before. This is often associated with epilepsy. There is a phenomenon that is related to depersonalisation called "derealisation". With derealisation, the person feels normal but objects seem distant and unreal even though they know that the surrounding objects are real. This may sometimes occur in combination with depersonalisation and, like it, passes quickly.

Cause Uncertain

The changes that occur in the brain are not fully established yet. Theories focus on the possibility of a disruption or imbalance in the part of the brain that regulates incoming stimuli with our sense of our self in the present. This part of the brain is referred to as the temporal lobe and one specific part, known as the amygdala, may be crucial.

Many people wonder if the feelings of detachment suggest some underlying lack of emotion in them for their family. However, these types of psychological explanations have not been shown to apply in depersonalisation. What may be important, however, is whether you are excessively tired at present or perhaps placing yourself under very severe stress.

Specialist Treatment

Whether you need to see a specialist depends on how often you have these experiences and how long they last. If they occur every few days and last for thirty to forty minutes then you should certainly ask to see a psychiatrist or a neurologist. However, if these episodes are fleeting and you have an explanation for them then you might try dealing with them yourself by resting, taking care not to drink alcohol, practising relaxation/meditation and eating a healthy diet, as these can influence the condition. If you feel you need reassurance then of course you should seek further advice also.

* * *

There is very little that can be done to treat this condition other than the practical measures I have already suggested and in the vast majority of people the episodes resolve spontaneously. When depersonalisation and derealisation are symptoms of underlying anxiety or depression, treating these will result in improvement. However, when the episodes occur spontaneously and without any obvious cause, and this is rare, there is little evidence that any specific treatment works. Even in these circumstances depersonalisation does not progress to anything more serious although it is indeed unpleasant.

Useful Reading

Camus, Albert, *The Outsider*, Penguin Modern Classics (A useful description of this condition, although the explanation offered is philosophical rather than medical)

Useful Website

www.benzo.org.uk
(Click on Symptoms and then click Depersonalisation and Derealisation)

I am twenty-two and I have recently started to feel very anxious, frightened and sweaty for no reason. These "attacks" come on without warning and happen once or twice each day. I am terrified that I will die as I feel dizzy and my heart thumps. I have even stopped going out in case I should get one when I am away from home. I have no particular problems in my life now or in the past yet I don't know what is the matter with me. What can I do?

You are describing classic panic attacks. These are overwhelming bursts of anxiety that usually occur for no reason and are accompanied by various unpleasant physical sensations like those you describe – palpitations, sweating and dizziness. Sometimes there is difficulty breathing and there may even be chest pain, so that the attack resembles a heart attack and many people mistakenly go to the emergency department. Whilst this may be a sensible precaution in the first instance, once there is confirmation that you do not have heart disease you should resist the temptation.

Common Fear

Panic attacks are common and 3–4 per cent of people experience them at some point in their lives. It is common for the sufferer to feel they are going to faint and, like you, to avoid going out lest the attack recur. The danger of this avoidance is that agoraphobia may develop, causing a further restriction in day-to-day activities and ultimately making the condition doubly difficult to treat.

Panic Disorder

From your description it is likely that you have a condition called panic disorder, since you say you do not have any particular personal problems and you do not mention any other symptoms such as sleep or appetite disturbance. Panic attacks can occur in a number of different emotional conditions including depressive illness, phobias (when they are closely linked to being in the feared situation), following bad trips on illicit drugs, during alcohol withdrawal and with hyperactivity of the thyroid gland in the neck.

Therapy

A useful emergency measure, should you get a panic attack and become very frightened, is to re-breath into a paper bag (not a plastic bag) and for the moment it might be worthwhile carrying one in your bag. However, you must see your general practitioner, who will carry out some simple tests to exclude any physical illness that could be causing the panic attacks. Once this has been done treatment can commence. It will only involve medication if the panic is so overwhelming that you cannot begin to control it yourself and it will then only be used in the short term, for a few weeks at most.

The first principle of non-drug treatment consists of distracting yourself from the symptoms when they occur. Relaxation tapes may be helpful or if you are too anxious to relax then you may find exercise a helpful alternative. It does not have to be very vigorous – going for a walk or a jog might refocus you. If you have noticed that coffee or alcohol contribute to your symptoms you should avoid these. Above all, you must not restrict your activities just to avoid a panic attack – this will allow your condition to control you rather than you mastering it.

Diary

Your general practitioner may refer you to a psychiatrist or psychologist for cognitive therapy. You will be asked to keep a diary of your symptoms and also of the frightening thoughts that occur with these. Many people get thoughts such as "I'm going to die" or "I will embarrass my friends" along with the uncomfortable symptoms. If you think about it, how many panic attacks have occurred during which you died or caused your friends to feel ashamed of you?! Your therapist will take you through all your negative thoughts in detail and you will come to appreciate that the fears you have around the symptoms are without foundation. They will diminish and eventually disappear, though treatment may take a few months.

* * *

Since panic attacks can be effectively treated I recommend that you pursue this sooner rather than later and learn to gain control over these distressing symptoms.

Useful Reading

Sheehan, Elaine (1996) *Anxiety: Phobias and Panic Attacks: Your Questions Answered*, Element Books: London

Useful Website

www.panicportal.com

I recently had a baby and since then I have become preoccupied by cleanliness. I was always very meticulous about hygiene but my husband says I have gone over the top. I sterilise the bottle four or five times and wash my hands several times after changing her nappy. I think these are just normal precautions but my husband says I need professional help.

It is difficult to say whether you need professional help. Many new mothers are overly concerned about cleanliness but as time goes by they learn to relax a little and recognise that within reason it is impossible to remove all risks of exposure to dirt. It really depends on how much time you spend on these habits. Do they interfere with your life? What is your reaction if you cannot carry them out? Do you just get a little tense but then continue with your usual routine or do you become very distressed so that controlling these urges becomes difficult? A further consideration is whether you have other fears of dirt that are unrelated to the baby: are you able to shake hands, open doors and touch objects that have been handled by others? If your concerns are only focussed on the baby you may just need to gain some confidence about what is safe and not safe for her.

Obsessive-Compulsive Disorder

There is a condition called obsessive-compulsive disorder (OCD) in which one of the concerns is dirt. Consequently, the person washes repeatedly, will have great difficulty touching objects that others have had contact with and often devotes hours every day trying to avoid contamination. Similar preoccupations can be found in depression and the possibility that you may have post-natal depression should also be explored with your doctor. I suggest that you visit your doctor, with your husband if possible, so that the full picture from your perspective and that of your husband can be presented.

Embarrassment

Many people think that these problems indicate they are "going mad" or they are too embarrassed to discuss them. Is it possible that you too are embarrassed by them? This should not deter you from seeking help, as habits such as these are relatively common and the doctor will be familiar with them. Sometimes there are other associated rituals such as checking doors repeatedly. Other people get thoughts that are distressing. For example, a woman may think of taking a child from a pram, others think about knives or get obscene words intruding into their everyday thoughts. Known as rumination, these thoughts or ideas are never acted upon, so if you are also experiencing these you do not need to fear that you will carry them out – you won't.

Self-Help

In helping yourself you should begin by gradually reducing the number of times you sterilise the bottle. Make a contract with yourself to stop after, say, two attempts and request that your husband helps you to achieve this by taking the bottle from you. Initially, you may find that your level of tension increases when this happens but, over time, it will be easier. Once you have successfully curbed your tendency to clean the bottle excessively you should move on to the next problem area, such as excessive hand washing. Again, you should force yourself to stop washing after one or two attempts, assisted by the restraining help of your husband.

***

If this is unsuccessful then you definitely should visit your doctor. The most likely causes are normal nervousness about hygiene that is part of being a new mother or OCD, and you may also have post-natal depression. Your doctor can help to identify the cause and, if necessary, recommend treatment.

Useful Reading

Toates, F. (1990) *Obsessional Thoughts and Behaviour*, Thorsons: London

Useful Websites

www.ocdcentre.com

www.nhsdirect.nhs.uk

I am twenty and have recently become preoccupied by cleanliness. It's not that my personal hygiene was ever poor, but in the past six months or so I have been showering about five times every day and I spend hours washing my hands, to the extent that they are red and raw. My parents say I had a spell like this as a child but that it passed after a few months. I am off college at present because my life is so taken up by these habits. Can I be helped?

It sounds as though you have a condition called obsessive-compulsive disorder, also termed OCD, and you can be helped. It is not uncommon for some people with this disorder to have a history of similar symptoms in childhood and for these to improve without treatment, as they did in your case.

Unfortunately, the word "obsession" is commonly used in everyday speech where it describes being excessively worried about some problem. In describing this disorder, however, the word has a different meaning and refers to a repetitive set of behaviours that the person often tries to resist, recognising them as senseless. They can be very incapacitating as they consume a lot of time. Shakespeare provides an example of OCD when he describes the hand-washing ritual of Lady Macbeth just before her death.

Progress

The advances made in understanding OCD are illustrative of the progress that has been made in our knowledge of the causes and treatment of mental health problems in general in the past decade. Until recently it was thought that this was a rare disorder. We now know that this is not so and it is found in 2–3 per cent of the general adult population. As well as hand-washing rituals, some people describe constantly checking doors and windows. Others get unpleasant and intrusive thoughts of numbers or words or images. These are known as ruminations. Obsessional behaviour around dirt and contamination such as you are experiencing are the most common.

Good News

In the past decade OCD has moved from being a very disabling and difficult condition to treat to being very treatment responsive. Freud believed that OCD was related to difficulties arising during the early years of life, but these psychoanalytic theories have been overturned by biological and X-ray studies that have shown changes in brain metabolism in an area of the brain known as the pre-frontal cortex.

The good news is that this is a treatable condition and there are very specific interventions that can help overcome the disorder to the extent that one can lead a normal life in every respect. The optimum treatment is a combination of behavioural treatment and medication. Although either alone may be effective in mild cases, the effects last longer with both in combination. Behaviour therapy is usually conducted in an out-patient setting and consists of developing strategies to reduce the frequency of the repetitive behaviour. It is useful to involve a close family member to assist you in practising some of the techniques. Before treatment begins families are often driven to despair by the behaviour and they find it reassuring to become engaged in treatment, with the sufferer's permission of course. You do not mention the impact your behaviour has had on your family but it must be significant as you are incapacitated enough to require time off college.

In the past five years some specific anti-obsessional drugs have been developed and these enhance treatment further. These are not addictive and although initial effects are seen after three to four weeks it takes up to four months before maximum benefit is achieved. Once remission occurs it is advisable to have "top-up" behaviour therapy sessions from time to time. Medication may be required in the long term but this will be a matter for discussion with your therapist.

* * *

You must consult your general practitioner immediately who should refer you to a psychiatrist. A behaviour therapist working in the psychiatrist's team will also see you. Although you are very troubled by your rituals at present you can look forward to getting back to college and to leading a normal life.

Useful Reading

De Silva, P. and Rachman, S. (1999) *Obsessive-Compulsive Disorder: The Facts*, Oxford University Press: Oxford

Useful Website

www.mindinfo.co.uk

I am thirty-five and extremely shy. I get very nervous when I have to meet strangers and I blush the minute they speak to me. I had a few friends at school but they have stopped asking me to go out and I rarely see them now. I would love to have a girlfriend and eventually get married but I cannot even pluck up the courage to ask a girl out. I have an office job but even there I avoid my workmates if I can. I just don't know what to do. Would counselling help?

You have a condition known as social anxiety (also called social phobia). It is quite common, probably affecting 3 per cent of the population according to figures from the US – there is no data available for Ireland. Sometimes the problem may not even be recognised as a condition requiring treatment and people with the condition are thought of as quiet, shy or even "snooty". However, your problem is much more than shyness, as it seems to be having a significant impact on your life.

Negative Effects

Not only is social anxiety associated with fear of meeting with and talking to people as you describe but some sufferers find it difficult to answer the telephone or stand in a queue. Some people cannot eat in public and even at home will chose to eat alone, away from everybody else. Difficulty speaking in public is another feature of the condition. Of course, not everybody has all of these difficulties and many of those with social phobia have problems in only one or two areas of life, with other aspects of life being normal. At its most severe, however, the individual is isolated and unable to make any friends or have any contact with strangers, to the extent that work becomes impossible. What is common to all sufferers is that there is intense self-consciousness, self-scrutiny and fear around new people.

Panic

The immediate effect of this fear is that the person will often experience a surge of fear and with it sweating, palpitations (thumping of the heart), dizziness and difficulty breathing. This intense fear then further fuels the pre-existing anxiety with the result that there may be increasing avoidance of social situations. Sometimes it feels as though a fainting episode will occur but this is a rare occurrence and generally the panic subsides. It is tempting to rush away from the anxiety-provoking situation and isolate oneself, as you are doing, but this will ultimately worsen the anxiety level overall. So, it is important to sit through the panic and fear rather than avoiding them.

Therapy

The good news is that social anxiety can be treated. The best treatment is cognitive-behaviour therapy. Counselling, by constantly focussing on feelings, would tend to worsen the self-consciousness with its emphasis on personal reflection. The aim of cognitive therapy is to bring about change by examining the faulty beliefs that underlie shyness. For example, shy people often believe that they are being critically examined by others or that they will make fools of themselves. They may also fear giving offence to others. The goal of cognitive therapy is to change these thoughts and replace them with more accurate self-evaluation.

Initially, treatment may be carried out on an individual basis until the person is ready for group interventions. Group therapy achieves the best results, since the condition is ultimately about how we respond to other people. Medication has little part to play unless the anxiety is so crippling that the talking therapy cannot even begin.

Techniques

In treatment you will firstly be taught to relax in social situations by using simple techniques to overcome tension. Then your thoughts about what people may be thinking when they meet you will be challenged. You will also be encouraged to rehearse meetings and social encounters before they happen. Many therapists video-tape the sessions to provide you with feedback on how you really perform in front of people, since people with social phobia often exaggerate their anxiety and awkwardness. You will also be given homework assignments to carry out in between sessions.

* * *

For the moment, you can help yourself by not avoiding the situations that make you anxious, if at all possible. You could also practise what you will say in advance of some social encounters, for example when you are introduced to a stranger. I suggest, however, that you also seek appropriate treatment as soon as possible.

Useful Reading

Butler, Gillian (1999) *Overcoming Social Anxiety and Shyness*, Robinson Publishing Ltd, London

Useful Websites

www.social-anxiety.org/

http://www.rcpsych.ac.uk/info/help/socphob/

Useful Contact

Out and About Organisation
140 St Lawrence's Road, Clontarf, Dublin 11, Tel. (01) 8338252

Anxiety Disorders

I am thirty and for many years I have been doing everything I can to avoid cats. It began when I was a child of eight and I don't know why. It is now a huge problem as most of my neighbours have cats and I have to cope with them every day. In addition, my children are begging me to get a kitten. I haven't told them of my fear because I think they might tease me about it. I feel I need to see a counsellor to get to the root cause. Can you help?

Your fear of cats seems to be a great inconvenience to you indeed. However, phobias such as yours are very common and all kinds of objects and animals may be the source of the fear, including spiders, thunder, wind, toilets and so on. Fear of cats is among the most commonly described.

The depth of the fear varies from those who, like you, do everything possible to avoid them to those who can tolerate them from a distance or can allow their children to keep pets provided they have no contact with them. Treatment can help you overcome this phobia but counselling to explore underlying causes, although intuitively seeming like a good idea, may not help rid you of this fear and in any event would take a very long time. You need to see a behaviour therapist.

Avoidance

It is understandable that you would do everything you can to avoid being near cats and although this will help control your anxiety at the time, it will ultimately worsen the fear. Then the next time you see a cat you will be even more frightened and a vicious circle will develop of increasing fear leading to further avoidance with even more fear on the next exposure. So the next time you see a cat you should stand and look at it for a while and you may find that your anxiety in that particular situation will reduce, perhaps after a few minutes.

Self-Help

There is a lot you can do for yourself to overcome this fear. Do not be tempted to expose yourself to too much fear initially. Instead, a gradual approach, known as graded exposure, will be more effective.

Firstly, you need to decide what you want to achieve – do you want to be able to hold a cat in your arms or would being able to have one as a pet but with no physical contact be sufficient? Then make a list of all the situations that cause you fear at present, from the least to the most terrifying. This is known as a hierarchy of fears. For example, looking at a picture of a cat may only cause mild anxiety but seeing one in your garden may be terrifying. This list may be quite long but it is crucial to spend time preparing it, since the principle of treatment is to expose yourself to each of these situations beginning with the mildest and working through them until you have reached the most frightening.

Beginning Exposure

You should begin by simply imagining yourself in the least anxiety-provoking situation and think about this until your level of fear diminishes. You should then carry out the behaviour in reality and remain in the situation until you are completely comfortable being there. Some people omit the exposure-in-imagination and proceed straight to real exposure. Several sessions may be required before you are calm enough to move on to the next item in the hierarchy.

Relax and Reward

Before you begin each session you should make sure that you are relaxed by listening to some restful music or by doing relaxation exercises. Also, avoid trying to "fit it in" during a busy schedule. If you are rushed or tense beginning each session it will take much longer to reduce your level of anxiety during exposure. Between sessions it is crucial that you practise and continually re-expose yourself to the various fear-inducing situations that you have overcome. If this does not happen the fear will return again rapidly. At the outset you should set yourself some targets and as you reach each one you can reward yourself by buying something for yourself or doing some activity that you enjoy.

Behaviour Therapy

I hope the above works for you. If it does not, you should consult your general practitioner, who will refer you to a behaviour therapist. Such therapists are often psychiatric nurses with special qualifications in that area or clinical psychologists who are employed by health boards throughout the country.

* * *

You will be comforted to know that most people with phobias can be successfully treated and can overcome their fear completely.

Useful Reading

Sheehan, Elaine (1996) *Anxiety: Phobias and Panic Attacks: Your Questions Answered*, Element Books: London

Marks, Isaac (2001) *Living with Fear*, McGraw Hill: London

Useful Websites

www.nomorepanic.co.uk

http://www.rcpsych.ac.uk/info/help/anxiety/

I am thirty-three and I was put on tranquillizers four years ago because of some personal problems. I had just got married and moved house to be near my husband's work. I also got a new job and although I tried to settle into my new life I found it very difficult and was worried all the time. I was unhappy at work and couldn't sleep. I have tried to come off these drugs but I get tense and irritable. My friends tell me to throw them down the sink!

Tranquillizers, known as benzodiazepines, can lead to physical dependence and the symptoms you describe when you try to stop them would suggest that, through no fault of your own, you have developed just such a dependence. This means that you have a physical need to keep taking them just to prevent the withdrawal symptoms that you describe. It is not that you are taking them to get high, as people do with drugs such as heroin or cocaine.

Many people are prescribed tranquillizers to help them deal with a period of "stress" in their lives and even when the problem has resolved the medication is inadvertently not discontinued. Ideally, tranquillizers should not be taken for longer than six weeks. It is also suggested that instead of being taken regularly they be taken only when symptoms are present that require them. This allows for drug-free periods and so minimises the risk of dependence.

Continuing Anxiety

One of the problems with these drugs is that the withdrawal symptoms are identical to the symptoms of anxiety and stress for which they were prescribed. This creates a vicious circle, as it is assumed that the continuing symptoms require ongoing treatment. The result is increasing use and increasing physical dependence.

You would be very foolish to throw away your tablets as your friends suggest, although I can understand why you might be tempted to do so. However, the withdrawal reaction can be serious and includes symptoms such as sleeplessness, tension, irritability and panic. Even more serious than those are the fits that sometimes occur and the feelings of detachment from oneself and from one's surroundings. These are termed depersonalisation and derealisation and can be very frightening. Sometimes there is also an increased sense of hearing.

Gradual Reduction

It is best to discontinue these drugs by a slight reduction in dose for two weeks and to continue at the new level until any withdrawal symptoms, which should be very mild – if present at all, have gone. The process can then be repeated until you are off all the medication.

There are two groups of benzodiazepine tranquillizers and it is important to find out if you are on the long- or short-acting variety, since withdrawal symptoms are more severe with the short-acting group. In fact, some people, under the supervision of their family doctor, change to a long-acting medication before attempting to discontinue them. Some doctors also cover the withdrawal period by prescribing an antidepressant so as to minimise withdrawal symptoms. This would of course be stopped once the withdrawal had concluded.

* * *

It is clear that discontinuing this group of drugs must be done under medical supervision. In addition, some family doctors run groups to assist in motivating and supporting those discontinuing these medications. You must remember that it will not happen overnight and it can take several months. Your motivation is crucial in having a successful withdrawal.

Useful Reading

Ling, W., Smith, D.E. and Wesson, D. (1994) *Prescription Drug Abuse and Addiction: Answering Your Questions*, Hazelden Publishing and Educational Services: USA

Useful Website

www.benzo.org.uk

I have recently had some problems with my boss and I dread going to work every day. I am having trouble sleeping, as I am constantly worried about work and about the arguments that will occur the following day. I feel tense all the time yet at the weekends I feel very relaxed. I have lost weight and feel tired all the time – as a result my work is suffering. My general practitioner has suggested I take tranquillizers for a short while but I am terrified as I hear they are very addictive.

It must be terrible for you having to face problems at work every day and it is hardly surprising that you are tense and nervous about it. This cannot continue, of course, and you should seek advice from the human resources department or, if that is unhelpful, from a solicitor if you feel it constitutes bullying or harassment. Meanwhile, your understandable tension and worry must be brought under control, as it seems to be affecting your health and your functioning generally.

Relaxation Tapes

There are some very good relaxation tapes on the market and they can be bought in many health shops or in some bookshops. Playing one of these at night may help you unwind. However, if your level of anxiety is very high you may not be able to distance yourself enough from your problems to concentrate on the tape or to benefit in any way.

Tranquillizers

Your general practitioner is correct in suggesting short-term tranquillizers as they will certainly be very effective in reducing your feelings of tension and they will help you to sleep, resulting in an overall improvement in your well-being. You are correct to have some reservations, since tranquillizers can cause dependence if taken for prolonged periods – four weeks is the recommended duration. Also, if your problems are likely to be long term you should be cautious, as you may not want to embark on the road of using medication instead of solving the real problem.

No Highs

The dependence caused by these medications, known as "minor" tranquillizers (to distinguish them from "major" tranquillizers, which are not addictive and are usually used for more serious psychiatric disorders such as schizophrenia), stems from the necessity to continue taking them to prevent withdrawal symptoms. They do not cause a "high" like other drugs of dependence such as heroin.

The most common tranquillizers are known as benzodiazepines and are divided into two groups – those that act quickly on symptoms and leave the body rapidly, known as short-acting tranquillizers, and the long-acting group that have a more prolonged action and are metabolised more slowly. The second group are less likely to be associated with withdrawal symptoms when they are discontinued, although they may take an hour or so to alleviate the symptoms for which they are prescribed. With either group you may feel drowsy or "hung over" in the morning and this may further deter you from taking them.

Prescriptions

Under new regulations, you will have to visit your general practitioner every month to obtain a new prescription rather than getting a supply for a few months as in the past. This may be inconvenient for you but the rule has been put in place to try to reduce the numbers of prescriptions for these drugs and ultimately the likelihood of dependence.

* * *

You may opt to take this medication in the short term, but this is not a long-term solution – really it is not a solution at all. You should seek advice as suggested above or look for alternative employment. You should also make use of your friends and work colleagues for support during this difficult time.

Useful Website

www.benzo.org.uk

My daughter was mugged on her way home from work recently. She has been terrified since and cannot stop talking or thinking about what happened. I have been reading a book about a kidnap victim who was debriefed afterwards. What is debriefing and I wonder should my daughter have received it? Would it have helped her cope better?

Psychological debriefing, sometimes called Critical Incident Stress Debriefing, is a relatively new form of treatment that has been used following serious and traumatic events. It was first described in 1983 when it was used to assist ambulance personnel in dealing with the distress associated with their work, such as seeing badly mutilated bodies after accidents. It has also been used for fire fighters and for soldiers after battle and most hospitals have incorporated this intervention into their major accident plans – in other words debriefing has become a mainstream intervention. Psychologists and psychiatrists have written about it extensively since the Gulf War, where soldiers and body-handlers witnessed horrifying sights. You may also have heard it mentioned on news bulletins, especially following kidnappings or hijackings. So mugging is the kind of traumatic incident for which it might until recently have been considered to have some value.

Preventing Problems

The thinking behind it is that the debriefing sessions help bring to full awareness the trauma that has been witnessed and that by releasing emotion surrounding the events serious psychological injury will be prevented. Those who promote debriefing are concerned that many people subjected to extreme trauma prefer to push it to the back of their minds and avoid speaking or even thinking about it, leading to serious psychological problems later.

The debriefing sessions vary in number but are usually no more than two or three, taking place a few days after the traumatic incident. Their duration is brief and lasts about two hours. During the session the person recounts the events in detail, and is encouraged to describe the fears and emotions associated with these. They are designed to facilitate the free expression of emotion.

Recent Research

Until recently there were few research studies to indicate whether this treatment was helpful or not, although, on the face of it, one would expect that it should be. The results of recent studies have been very surprising. They have shown that not only is debriefing not helpful, but that those given this intervention are at greater risk of later emotional problems than those not given this

Anxiety Disorders

treatment. This unexpected finding has lead to recommendations that compulsory debriefing of army personnel who have witnessed terrifying events should be abandoned. The explanation for these worrying results is that the natural healing process is interrupted and so, like a wound that is beginning to heal, the debriefing acts like a needle prising open the wound again.

This is not to say that if your daughter is very distressed and needs help she should be deprived of it. However, the therapist would have to decide on whether her feelings were more severe than might be expected following such a frightening incident – indeed it would be abnormal not to be distressed. Usually following a mugging, the fear, crying and sleep problems might take several weeks to improve and rehearsing what has happened over and over again might prolong her upset.

If her symptoms do continue then some intervention to help her overcome the fear might be necessary. If she continues to avoid the place where the incident occurred, she should be seen by a behaviour therapist, who will gradually "expose" her to these feared situations and places. This may involve rehearsing a visit in her imagination until her fear had greatly reduced followed by gradually approaching the place under the guidance of her therapist.

* * *

Your daughter may well be fortunate in not having sought debriefing as there is a possibility that her symptoms might be even more severe than they are now.

Useful Reading

Kinchin, D. (1994) *Post-Traumatic Stress Disorder: A Practical Guide to Recovery*, Thorsons: London

Useful Website

www.ncptsd.org

Useful Contact

Victim Support
29 Dame Street, Dublin 2, Tel. (01) 6798673

Bereavement

Grief can't be shared. Everyone carries it alone, his own burden, his own way.

Anne Morrow Lindbergh,
Dearly Beloved, *1962*

Bereavement

My mother died suddenly about six months ago. She was seventy. I am still devastated by the loss. She was my best friend and lived with us. I can't stop crying and I can't even think about going to the grave or giving away her clothes. Will this sadness ever go away? My husband and family tell me that things will get better but I can't believe that.

I am sorry that your mother has died. It is very difficult when the death is sudden and when one is so close. There is no time to prepare or to say goodbye. However, you can take comfort from the reality that almost everybody, with the exception of those who are very vulnerable, get over such a loss. That is not to say that they do not still miss the loved one but the crying, the terrible sense of loneliness and the longing to see or speak to the person again all diminish with time.

Vulnerable

The vulnerable people who have trouble coming to terms with bereavement are those who were very dependent on their parents emotionally, for help and advice, or those with learning problems who are unable to express their fear of being left without anybody to love and care for them. In addition, those who do not have outside support or whose only emotional tie is with their parents would also have trouble coming to terms with death. Since you were so close to your mother, it may take you longer than usual to deal with the loss. However, I do not think that you have the same level of vulnerability as I have just mentioned and your husband and family seem to be loving and caring.

Healing

I realise that it will be difficult but you must consider visiting the grave, as that will help you truly accept that your mother is gone. The longer you avoid it the harder it will get. You might want to take a friend or family member with you so that you do not feel so alone, though sometimes people wish to be alone with their loved one for that first visit. You may feel that if you cry, you won't be able to stop. There is no need to feel this way as crying is an essential part of grieving that will ultimately allow your sorrow to heal. It will also help if you look at photographs of your mother and yourself so that you can bring back memories of the happy times you spent together. This will upset you but crying is what you need to do at present.

Many people talk to their deceased loved ones and get comfort from that, feeling that they are in contact and that they are being "looked after". This is not a sign of instability as some people think; it indicates normal grieving. Talking about your mother and the things you remember fondly about her will also help you to disengage gradually from her. You must also consider giving away some of your mother's possessions, but be sure to keep some mementos. Perhaps this is premature, but it will have to be faced when you feel able. In due course, you will have to redecorate her bedroom. When you have achieved this you will indeed have "moved on" in your grief.

You should also find things to do that give you pleasure, even if for only a brief period. Going for a walk, returning to your hobbies or watching a favourite TV programme will help take you out of your sadness and temporarily act as a distraction so that you do not become entrapped in sadness. None of this means that you will forget her or that your love for her will diminish – it will just change.

Professional Help

You may want to consider bereavement counselling if you are not beginning to come to terms with her death after a few months. This would give you the freedom to cry and say what you want about your mother and her death. The counsellor will proceed at your pace only and there will be no set timetable. Sometimes it may take no more than a few weeks; other times it may take several months.

* * *

If your sadness continues you must definitely visit your doctor, since depression can complicate grief. If you are still crying, not sleeping, getting little pleasure from life and very bound up with your loss, then it is possible you have developed a clinical depression, which your doctor can treat. You can take consolation that even in these circumstances, peace and contentment does return.

Useful Reading
Keneally, Christy, (1999) *Life after Loss*, Mercier Press: Cork

Useful Website
http://www.rcpsych.ac.uk/info/help/bereav/

My husband, aged fifty-eight, died a few months ago. It was very sudden and since I got the terrible news I have no feeling at all. I went to the funeral but I never cried and I have been on "autopilot" since then. I feel numb and cut-off and I am unable to visit the grave, although my family encourage me to go. I just can't believe my husband is dead. Christmas was dreadful and I began to cry at midnight Mass but stopped myself. I just don't know what to do. Would bereavement counselling help?

I am sorry that you have lost your husband – it must have been a terrible shock for you. When bad news is delivered, as the unexpected, sad news about your husband was, this feeling of numbness is common. Usually, however, it disappears after a short time, a few hours at most. In your case, this feeling of numbness means that you are "stuck" in your grief and unable to progress to the next phase and overcome it. Bereavement counselling may be of great benefit to you, but there are also some things you can do for yourself that might avoid the need for outside help. Indeed, the fact that you began to cry at Christmas is a sign that you may be beginning to move in your grief, so you must not stop yourself from crying when the urge comes.

Rituals

You were absolutely right to go to the funeral, even though you felt cut-off and detached. If you had not gone, you would have been storing up further problems for yourself. However, you must now visit the grave also. The reason for your reluctance at present is probably because you do not want to admit that your husband really is gone forever. In a sense, the numb feeling is protecting you emotionally from this realisation, although it is a false protection. The sooner you recognise that your husband has died the sooner you will begin to grieve normally. As a first step in that process, you must regularly visit the grave.

Some people feel exposed if the visit is with a family member or friend, so going there on your own would give you the space to cry and grieve. However, you may want a family member or friend with you for support – you could ask them to wait in the car while you have your own time by the graveside. There is no need to feel afraid of your tears – they will be tears of sadness as well as of healing. Once you start to cry, the numb feeling will disappear.

Reminders

It helps also if you look at photographs of your husband and yourself and bring back memories of the happy times you spent together. This will upset you but crying is what you need to do at present. Many people talk to their deceased relatives and get comfort from that, feeling that they are in contact and that they are being "looked after". This is not a sign of instability as people often fear, but is an indicator of normal grieving. Talking about your husband, and the things he did or said with family members may also help you to disengage gradually from him.

You do not indicate if you have given away his clothes yet, but that is something you will have to consider also, in due course. You must keep a few mementos and carrying something that you particularly associated with him such as a pen or handkerchief will ease this painful process as well as give you the comfort of feeling part of him with you.

Mixed Emotions

Grief is complicated and emotions are often very mixed with feelings of emptiness and sadness intermixed with anger at being left behind, especially if there are financial or other problems for you to deal with. With time, these will disappear but acknowledging them in the first place is helpful. However, they should not take over and you need to remind yourself of the good times. Your sadness at Christmas may mark the beginning of the end of your grief and you should cry whenever you feel the need rather than trying to avoid this. If you do not cry your grief will continue and this may lead to other emotional problems such as depression.

* * *

Hopefully you will progress from the past to the future and when this happens you must not feel guilty as some people do. Moving on from your overwhelming numbness or sadness while living with the fond memories is what healing is all about.

Useful Reading

Kenneally, Christy (1999) *Life after Loss*, Mercier Press: Cork

Useful Website

http://www.rcpsych.ac.uk/info/help/bereav/

I am so angry since my mother died a few weeks ago. She took her own life. She had often threatened it in the past, especially when she was depressed. She had been under a psychiatrist for years yet he was unable to prevent this. I feel that she did a cowardly thing and I hate her doctors for not being able to stop her. Part of me is very guilty because I feel a sense of relief. Is there anything I can do to move on from this tragedy?

Firstly, I would like to express my sympathy to you on your mother's death. Even after a long illness it is always a time of great sorrow, and suicide is especially upsetting. It would be naive of me to tell you how you should feel, since you are currently experiencing the gamut of emotions that any person might feel in these circumstances, and you know too well the intensity of these.

Despair

Suicide is often perceived as an act of escape and cowardice to those left behind but it is important to realise that the person driven to suicide is in absolute despair. Whilst it may seem an easy option it stems from a profound sense of hopelessness, which is a deeply distressing emotion to feel. It has been described by some in spiritual terms and St John of the Cross wrote about it in his work *The Dark Night of the Soul.* You are left behind struggling to pick up the pieces and to move forward. It is not surprising that you see your mother's action in this negative way.

Anger

While anger can occur even when death is expected, it is all the more likely to be a prominent feeling when death is unexpected and by the victim's own hand. This anger will pass as time goes by. When you are less raw you may experience the death of your mother as a sadness and a loss rather than something to be angry about. Your anger at the doctors is understandable and I suggest that you make contact with the psychiatrist in order to discuss your mother's death and the circumstances leading to it. It may throw another light on her death if, for example, she was refusing treatment or not taking her medication. If you have reason to believe that proper care was not given to your mother or that she was treated incorrectly then you have good reason to be angry and you need to inform the doctors of this so that, at least, it is not repeated with somebody else. Guilt is also part of the normal grieving process and you should not punish yourself for this feeling.

Grieving and Healing

People are helped to heal in various ways and for many the simple passage of time is enough. Gradually, you will feel these emotions lessen and you will begin to see beyond what has happened. Others find suicide support groups very helpful, since it is possible to meet and identify with the emotions experienced by others. Above all, you have to look after yourself and if there are people telling you that you should be going out, or going on holiday etc. take no notice. You need time and space and you are the person who knows best when to move on.

As in any bereavement, you should visit the grave, talk about your mother to family members or friends, even if for the moment it is in anger. Look at her photograph and talk to her also – tell her how you are feeling, both in yourself and about what she has done. You may even find it helpful to "write" to her.

* * *

Coming to terms with what has happened is painful and will possibly take longer than any other bereavement you have experienced. But do not give up; you will heal.

Useful Reading

McCarthy, Sarah (2001) *A Voice for those Bereaved by Suicide*, Veritas: Dublin

Useful Contact

The Samaritans
(Runs support groups for those bereaved by suicide)
Tel. (01) 8727700

I have just come out of hospital following a miscarriage. Although the pregnancy was unplanned I am now devastated by the loss. I have two children already and my husband and I had told them about the pregnancy. I am crying all the time and I feel guilty about not being happy with the pregnancy initially. My friends tell me I am lucky that I can become pregnant again.

I am so sorry that you have had a miscarriage. It is understandable that you are upset by the loss of the baby. Even when a pregnancy is not planned many are surprised by the power of the emotion that a miscarriage can bring. You were beginning to accept the pregnancy and perhaps you were having dreams and making plans already, even in a preliminary way, for the baby and your enlarged family. The fact that you had told your children shows that the baby you were carrying was already being accepted as part of that family.

Guilt

It is also understandable that you feel guilty that by not being very happy about the pregnancy initially you may in some way have caused this to happen. I am sure you know logically that this could not be the case, even though your heart tells you otherwise. There is certainly no research to suggest that miscarriages are more common in those who have unexpected pregnancies as distinct from those that are planned. For now, I think you should not be so hard on yourself and just accept that what has happened was a chance occurrence. You may also be seeking reassurance from your husband about this. I doubt that at present you will accept what he says but, in time, you will get a different perspective on things.

Time Out

You should if possible take more time for yourself at this point. Unfortunately, when a miscarriage occurs there is little time to prepare and often little warning. Our emotions thus become confused and muddled and many women describe leaving hospital in a confused and dazed state. Not surprisingly you are thinking about your baby and for now this is the right thing to do. Some women give their baby a name and even have a religious ceremony or commemoration to mark this life that has ended so early. Do not fight the thoughts and images of your baby but as they become less frequent you must not feel guilty either, as this is nature's way of healing your wounds.

It is very insensitive of others to remind you that you can become pregnant again, as it undermines your sadness at the loss of this baby, although I am sure they are well meaning. Perhaps you feel angry with them and this is another reason to take a bit more time off work just now.

Reminders

Many women find reminders of the baby difficult to deal with, particularly when friends become pregnant or are due to have babies around the time their baby was expected. At present, you may also find that even seeing baby clothes is very upsetting. However, as time goes by, especially once the date when your baby was due has passed, you will probably feel much better. If your sadness persists you should visit your doctor, as professional help may be needed to help you deal with the loss.

* * *

You may be tempted to become pregnant immediately and this is perfectly understandable. I suggest that you take a few months to grieve and when you are feeling stronger emotionally and physically you could, if you still wished, consider another pregnancy without any fear that you would be "replacing" the baby that you have lost. Then you will have a new and different baby worthy of love as a separate human being.

Useful Reading

Ingram, K.J. (1997) *Always Precious in our Memory: Reflections after Miscarriage, Stillbirth or Neonatal Death*, ACTA Publications (available from Amazon)

Useful Website

www.opendoors.com.au/EffectsMiscarriage

I am thirty-two and had an abortion four years ago after a brief relationship, which I knew was going nowhere. I went to England for the operation at fourteen weeks and I felt great relief afterwards. However, whenever the issue is debated I become very upset and feel so lonely and isolated. My friends tell me to forget about the past and get on with life – that I made the right decision at the time. I feel I made the wrong decision and I wish I could live my life over again. Can you help?

Unfortunately, many people try to get on with life by putting unpleasant thoughts and memories out of their mind. This can be effective, but only in the short term and it can be very hard work at times. Then when a reminder pops up the memory returns and because it has never been dealt with emotionally it becomes very distressing.

Relief and Regret

What you have described is characteristic of the reaction that many women have to abortion. There is initial relief, sometimes followed by a surge of gloom and guilt and finally a coming to terms with what has happened. Reminders of what has happened are a cause of great distress for many and some women become distressed when friends have babies or when they read about childbirth in magazines. In some instances, the regret never leaves entirely but the person is enabled to get on with life, as they confront their emotions.

Grief Undermined

Sometimes well-meaning friends and family are in fact unhelpful. Telling you that you should forget about what has happened is like telling a recently bereaved person to forget about their loved one. Your friends should acknowledge your sadness and allow you the space to speak of your grief. I am not surprised that you feel lonely if you have nobody to turn to who is willing to acknowledge how you feel. Part of the problem may be that they do not know how to react.

Acknowledge the Pain

You can do some things to help yourself such as crying and confronting your feelings, including those of guilt. These feelings must be acknowledged and accepted but they must not consume you. You cannot, as you say, turn back the clock, but you could help overcome your guilt by making "restitution" by, for example, giving some money to a suitable children's charity. Some women in these circumstances also find it helpful to have a private commemoration ceremony to acknowledge the baby – others even give a name to the baby. Putting your thoughts and feelings in writing can be immensely helpful, especially if you have nobody to talk to or if you find it difficult to discuss certain aspects of the abortion. There is no absolutely right response to your predicament and you should do whatever you feel best helps you.

Professional Help

If these simple measures do not help you should seek professional help. There are now several agencies offering counselling to those who have post-abortion difficulties. If you are religious you may find it helpful to speak to a priest or minister.

* * *

Although the memory of what has happened cannot be erased you will be able to come to terms with the situation if you now take the time to deal with it.

Useful Reading

Spencer, Catherine (1997) "Obstinate Questionings: An Experience of Abortion" in Angela Kennedy (ed.) *Swimming Against the Tide*, Open Air Publishing: Dublin

Useful Contact

CURA
Freephone 1850 62 26 26

My best friend's husband has just died by suicide and as she has no extended family I feel I must be there to help her. I just don't know how to respond. The funeral was a few days ago and she seems to be just getting on with life as if nothing had happened. I tried talking to her about the suicide but she refused and has hinted that it may have been an accident. I am so worried for her and for her teenage children. Can you give me some information?

This is indeed a terrible burden that you have to bear on behalf of your friend. As you realise, death by suicide is devastating for everybody concerned – family, friends, neighbours and for the whole community. Reactions to death by suicide are always profound, lengthy and comprised of complex emotions for all touched by it.

Mixed Emotions

Many people experience anger, guilt and even relief when a loved one takes their life. The anger may be directed at the person who has died and left them behind to deal with the loss. Others are angry with doctors and all the professionals who cared for the person that they did not prevent the death. Sometimes this may result in litigation for negligence.

Surprisingly, research has found that about 10 per cent of those bereaved by suicide feel relief that it has now happened, particularly among those who have been coping with the threat of suicide due to severe mental illness or drug abuse for many years. It may be that your friend is experiencing a greater tranquillity than ever before, especially if her husband had longstanding mental health problems, which might explain her calmness at present. Alternatively, she may be actively trying to put the death and the manner of his dying to the back of her mind. This is not helpful to her and, ultimately, she will have to confront her grief.

Guilt and Denial

The overwhelming emotion, however, is guilt: guilt that goodbyes could not be said, guilt that signs and signals of impending suicide were not identified or acted upon and self-blame that minor frictions in the family may have lead to the suicide. Some deny that the death was suicide at all and act upon the conviction that it was an accident, as your friend may be doing. You should not go along with this. However, although you could gently point out the truth to her, this may impair her relationship with you. You may find it better to avoid confrontation about this for the moment, though you should not agree with her either if she says the death was accidental, as this would re-enforce her false belief. Hopefully in her own time and space she will accept the reality of her husband's suicide. She will then strive to make sense of why he took his life and will be left sifting the good from the not-so-good memories. If she and her husband had a particularly close or a very poor relationship, her grief will be more protracted.

Children

If your friend does not accept the manner of her husband's death, it is possible that she will try to enmesh her children in her beliefs about his death also. However, as teenagers it is very likely that they have a full realisation of the manner of his death and they could be emotionally damaged if they are not allowed to establish their own acceptance of what has happened. So, even if their mother cannot speak to them about their father's tragic death, you should be prepared to do so, if they want or need you to. They too will be experiencing similar mixed feelings about the death of their father.

Practical Help

The assistance of family and friends is crucial following any death, but especially so following suicide when family members are hurting in a very profound way. Sometimes once the funeral is over friends get on with their lives – but that is the time when support and practical help is most needed.

You may be tempted to speak to your friend about his death being brave, or conversely a selfish act. There is no room for the moral high ground, no question of justifying what happened, only the reality of your friend being left with a loss and a pain like no other.

The support of others similarly bereaved is often most helpful following suicide. You may want to encourage your friend to go to such a group when the immediate shock is over, provided she is accepting that her husband's death was indeed by suicide.

***

Remember that you are not a professional but a friend. Use your instincts for compassion and kindness in helping your friend at this very sad time.

Useful Reading

McCarthy, Sarah (2001) *A Voice for those Bereaved by Suicide*, Veritas: Dublin

Jamison, Kay Redfield (1999) *Night Falls Fast: Understanding Suicide*, Vintage Books: New York

Useful Contact

The Samaritans
(Runs post-suicide support groups and can be contacted through the local organisations)
Tel. (01) 8781822 (Irish Regional Office)

Dementia

Dementia is not a natural part of ageing.

John Bayley,
husband of late Dame Iris Murdoch,
at launch of World Alzheimer Day, 2001

Dementia

I took my mother to the doctor recently as she was getting very forgetful. She is seventy and I was relieved when I was told that she did not have Alzheimer's disease. However, I was very upset when she had investigations and dementia due to narrowing of the arteries was discovered. Can you give me more information on this? Is there any cure?

I am sorry that your mother has this condition, which is known medically as vascular dementia or multi-infarct dementia. Unlike Alzheimer's disease, about which a lot has been written in the general press, there is much less public information about vascular dementia.

It is caused by narrowing of the blood vessels supplying oxygen to the brain and as a result of this brain tissue becomes damaged. Sometimes there may be mini-strokes and afterwards the memory changes become obvious. Those with high blood pressure or those with disease to the heart valves are at highest risk. The symptoms are generally the same as in Alzheimer's disease except that the deterioration in memory tends to occur in a step-wise manner rather than in the gradual way that is found in Alzheimer's disease. In other words, you may notice that the slight deterioration in your mother's memory will be static for months and then there will be another fall-off, which will remain unchanged for a further period. Changes to mood, especially depression, are common also.

Stable Symptoms

Since the pattern of this illness is stepwise with periods of stability in between, the person can adjust to the slight impairments in memory in the early stages. In addition, there is much less likely to be a change in personality in vascular dementia than there is in Alzheimer's disease and so the person is much more "themself".

Since a number of factors can contribute to vascular dementia, any changes to these will slow down the progress of the condition also. In a general way, a healthy diet and regular exercise may be helpful. In particular, if cholesterol or blood lipids are high these can worsen the blood vessel narrowing. Obesity may also add to this, so if your mother is overweight she should be strongly encouraged to loose weight. Illnesses such as diabetes mellitus, heart disease, a tendency to have blood clots, high blood pressure and alcohol abuse also worsen the condition due to their effect on blood vessels. Adequate treatment of these, if your mother has any of them, is vital: although it will not reverse damage already done, it may halt or slow the progress of the illness.

Memory Enhancers

There are treatments for improving memory in those with Alzheimer's disease and these are increasingly used in vascular dementia with varying results. It is certainly worth discussing them with your doctor and trying a course of them. There is also a practice of prescribing aspirin for this condition, since it reduces the risk of blood clots. However, the scientific evidence for its benefits in vascular dementia is lacking. If mood disturbance occurs then antidepressants may be necessary and if agitation or restlessness is prominent, as is common as the disease progresses, these are treated symptomatically with tranquillizers.

* * *

It must be upsetting and daunting for you to know that your mother has dementia. You should discuss the long-term care of your mother with other family members, if possible, and investigate various options with your doctor. Your mother may need the assistance of the geriatric team in your nearest hospital and a referral there is probably a good idea, in order to treat any underlying medical problems that may be contributing to her dementia. In due course, respite or even permanent care for your mother may need to be considered and you should also contact the Alzheimer society, which is a great source of support for carers of those with all types of dementia.

Useful Website

www.alzscot.org/info/vasculardementia.html

Useful Contact

Alzheimer Society of Ireland
(National helpline) 1800 341 341

Dementia

My uncle, aged sixty-eight, is an alcoholic and he has become very confused recently. I wonder could he be developing Alzheimer's disease. He lives near me so I see him most days. He has been talking about going to England to work and says that he has a wife there, although he has never lived outside this country. What should I do?

If your uncle is an alcoholic he may have one of several problems causing this confusion and he should visit his general practitioner so as to clarify the diagnosis. He may indeed be developing Alzheimer's disease, since he is of an age when this can occur. However, those who are alcoholic are no more prone to this than is anybody else but they can suffer from brain damage as a result of excessive alcohol intake.

Alcoholic Dementia

Many people do not know that alcohol itself is directly damaging to the brain and persistent abuse can cause dementia, not dissimilar to Alzheimer's disease. This is termed alcoholic dementia and unlike Alzheimer's disease it is not progressive – if the alcohol intake is brought under control the dementia remains static. This is a relatively common condition among people like your uncle who are alcohol dependent. For some reason, it is more commonly found among women than men, probably because women tend to drink at home and in secret and will therefore have a longer drinking history by the time the problem comes to light. Overall, those who drink heavily on a regular basis are more at risk than occasional binge drinkers. It can also develop over a short period of time if the alcohol intake is high enough.

Confabulations

There is also a form of brain damage due to alcohol abuse in which the person, like your uncle, makes up stories to fill in the gaps in their memory. These false tales are known as "confabulations" and it sounds as though your uncle's claim that he worked in England may be such an example. In addition, there will be loss of recent memory although long-term memory, i.e. memories of events from the past, remain intact. The condition itself is called Korsakoff's psychosis and like alcoholic dementia it remains static provided the alcohol abuse stops.

This form of alcohol-related damage is caused by a vitamin deficiency in the diet and it tends to occur after withdrawal from alcohol when vitamin stores have dropped. This is due to the effect that alcohol has on vitamin absorption and it can be prevented by supplementing the diet with vitamin

B1, known as thiamine. The deficiency results in small haemorrhages to certain parts of the underside of the brain.

Frontal Lobe Dementia

Many people who drink to excess are involved in accidents and fall a lot. They may physically damage their brains as a result of the impact of the fall, which causes swelling and scarring of brain tissue. The front of the brain, known as the frontal lobe, is concerned with judgement and self-control. The frontal lobe can also be damaged by alcohol, resulting in uncontrollable outbursts of aggressive behaviour as well as a decline in memory. Part of the brain at the back, called the cerebellum, can be damaged resulting in poor co-ordination of the hands and legs and dizziness. This may lead to problems walking and with balance.

Diagnosis

This can only be done by detailed neuro-cognitive assessment. This means referral to a clinical psychologist who can give tests of memory and of understanding. Abnormalities in these can point to the area of the brain that is damaged. A scan of the brain would also be very beneficial, although brain damage has to be quite marked before it will be discernable on a scan.

* * *

I am sorry that I cannot be more positive, but the crucial thing now is for your uncle to remain alcohol free. At his age, unlike younger people who have some possibility of recovery due to the greater re-generative powers of brain cells, it is unlikely that the present damage will improve, although its progress can be halted.

Useful Reading

Alcohol our Favourite Drug, Royal College of Psychiatrists, Public Education Department: London

Useful Website

www.betterhealth.vic.gov

Useful Contacts

Alcoholics Anonymous
109 South Circular Road, Dublin 8, Tel. (01) 4538998

Alcoholism Treatment Centre
Stanhope Street, Dublin 7, Tel. (01) 6673965

My brother is fifty-two and he has been complaining of memory loss. His wife died recently and he has found it very difficult to cope without her. Since her death nine months ago, I have begun to notice this change in him. He seems sad and forgets simple things like buying the groceries. He is just about managing to work but his workmates tell me they too have seen a great change in him. I am terrified that he may have Alzheimer's disease.

While memory loss is one of the features of Alzheimer's disease, there are many other more common causes. In particular, when somebody has a lot of worries they become distracted by them and ultimately appear forgetful. Depressive illness is also a common cause of forgetfulness, again due to lapses in concentration. The loss of memory in some people with depression is so severe that it resembles Alzheimer's disease or other types of dementia. This is called pseudodementia, since it resembles true dementia except that the memory loss is reversible and there is no damage to brain tissue as in the true dementias. Since your brother lost his wife recently it may be that it is his grief at her loss that is causing the poor memory, as he may have tipped into a depression requiring specific treatment.

Medical Attention

The only way to identify the cause is to insist that your brother visits his doctor. It would be helpful if you went with him also to inform the doctor of the extent of the memory loss. If the doctor feels that the memory loss is more than just ordinary forgetfulness he may then arrange for your brother to see a specialist for further investigations. A psychiatrist or psychologist may become involved in order to rule out common causes of memory loss, such as depression. Detailed memory testing may be required and will be carried out by a psychologist over a period of a few weeks. These tests take several hours to administer; they will identify the extent of the memory loss and possible causes. They also take into account the prior intelligence of the person and can be used irrespective of the educational background of the person – they are equally helpful in those who have university degrees as in those who left school at the age of fourteen. A brain scan may be carried out in order to complete the tests.

Causes

If no physical brain disease is found to underlie the memory loss then other causes such as anxiety and depression will be considered and treatment offered.

The memory loss will then improve and your brother should return to his prior level of functioning. If there is a physical cause such as Alzheimer's disease or some other dementia the treatment may vary and will depend on the diagnosis.

High blood pressure or high cholesterol can damage brain tissue and cause memory loss, and treatment of these will certainly improve memory. This is known as atherosclerotic dementia. Alcohol abuse can cause brain damage. In the early stages this is reversible, but later the damage is permanent. Discontinuing alcohol is imperative to prevent further deterioration. If the cause is Alzheimer's disease, there is no cure at present, though there are medications that are very helpful in improving the memory in the early stages of the disease.

Practical Help

At a practical level, it is important that your brother takes steps to minimise his forgetfulness, such as making lists and having reminders on his coffee table and in the kitchen. He should also avoid alcohol for the moment and make sure his diet is balanced, as a poor diet can cause memory impairment in some rare instances. There may be a temptation to delay seeking medical help for the moment in the hope that things will improve or simply to avoid the possibility that it cannot be cured. This would be foolish, since your brother may well have a reversible cause for his memory loss and it would be wrong to deprive him of the benefits of treatment. If there is no treatment then he and his family will need to make long-term plans to deal with this.

* * *

I hope that everything works out for your brother.

Useful Reading

Gidely, I. and Shears, R. (1989) *Alzheimer's: What It Is, How to Cope*, Unwin: North Sidney, Australia

Useful Website

www.alz.co.uk/alzheimers

Depression and Manic-Depression

Everybody gets depressed sometime.

Common myth

Depression and Manic-Depression

I hear and read a lot about depression but I don't really know what it is. The doctor has recently diagnosed my sister with it and I want to help her. Surely everyone gets depressed sometimes and really we should accept that it is nothing more than something that we all experience. Perhaps if my sister accepted it, it would go away.

You are right in some respects – everybody does feel depressed and low in mood from time to time. Indeed, it is quite normal to be down if we are bereaved, having personal problems or physically ill. This type of mood passes as time goes by or as the problems resolve. Doctors would not call this depression illness but might use the term "stress" to describe it.

Clinical Depression

When doctors speak of depression they are referring to a condition colloquially called clinical depression or depressive illness. This is different from the ordinary understandable gloom and sadness that you mention. It is unfortunate that the same words are used to describe each mood state, since one does not usually require any professional help whilst the other can be incapacitating and have a major impact on day-to-day life if not treated. Among the symptoms to watch out for are sleep problems, especially waking early in the morning, loss of appetite, feeling worse just after getting up, panic attacks and gloomy thoughts about death, about the past and feeling hopeless about the future. Spells of crying for no reason are common also, although if the depression is very severe the sufferer may not be able to cry at all and may even feel suicidal.

Pleasant Events

One of the key differences is that clinical depression, such as your sister has, does not go away when we go on holiday or have nice things happen to us. One would expect that positive events following on from unpleasant episodes should make us happy, but in clinical depression this does not happen, or if it does the effect is short lived, lasting only a few days or sometimes only a few hours. In some situations, a reaction that starts as "stress" following, say, a bereavement, tips over into a clinical depression and the low mood gets its own momentum. However, some 40 per cent of those with depressive illness have no trigger and may even search, in vain, in their past for some cause.

A Common Condition

Clinical depression is a relatively common condition effecting about 5–7 per cent of the population and the lifetime risk is around 30 per cent. It is much more common among women than men. Contrary to the myth, it is not more common at the time of the menopause but during the late 20s and into the 30s. The reason for the excess among women and in relatively young age groups is unclear at present. It is also more common in urban than rural areas.

Treatable

On a positive note, clinical depression is very treatable and the general practitioner can treat most sufferers without referring them to a psychiatrist. Your sister was quite right to contact her doctor when she was feeling "down"; tolerating it would not have been in her best interests. She is very likely to require antidepressants initially and if she has background problems that have triggered it she may need psychological help. Her doctor will be the best person to advise her on all aspects of her illness.

* * *

It is best if you are there to support her when she wants to talk with you, but also that you encourage her to take whatever treatment is prescribed or recommended. She will get better and you can give her hope through your positive attitude.

Useful Reading

Salmans, S. (1997) *Depression: Questions You Have, Answers You Need*, Thorsons: London

Useful Website

www.rcpsych.ac.uk
(Click on Mental Health Information and then follow the instructions)

Useful Contact

AWARE
72 Lower Leeson Street, Dublin 2, Tel. (01) 6617211

Depression and Manic-Depression

My general practitioner has recently told me that I have a depressive illness and that I need to take antidepressants. I do not want this, as I am fearful of becoming "hooked". My cousin is on antidepressants and has been unable to come off them. Also, I am frightened that I will be like a zombie and unable to work and I understand that the side effects are dreadful. Could I go for counselling instead?

Your general practitioner is correct in that if you have a depressive illness you do need an antidepressant or the illness could continue indefinitely. This would have a serious impact on your work, your family and your wider relationships. You should seriously consider antidepressants.

Antidepressants and Tranquillizers

Antidepressants are not addictive. When doctors speak of addiction they mean that there are withdrawal symptoms, that there is a necessity to increase the dose over time in order to achieve the same effect and often there is a craving. Antidepressants do not have these properties. They have been available for almost forty years and research suggests that addiction/dependence is not a problem.

Antidepressants and tranquillizers are often confused: it is the latter that are associated with dependence. Some people who take antidepressants, such as your cousin, cannot discontinue them as their illness recurs and the tablets are necessary to prevent a relapse. This is sometimes confused with dependence.

Side Effects

The side effects of antidepressants that you are fearful of vary and depend on the particular compound that you are taking. The older drugs, called the tricyclic antidepressants, may cause constipation, dry mouth and blurring of vision. They can cause drowsiness (which on the positive side will help you sleep). If you are drowsy by day or cannot tolerate the side effects then either the dose or the drug itself can be changed. It is important to realise that you may not experience any side effects. Newer antidepressants known as the SSRIs may cause headache and nausea. Some can cause a reduction in sexual interest and you may not want to eat as much as before. Again, if the side effects are a problem your doctor can adjust your treatment. You will not be a zombie and most people can work normally when taking this treatment. You may have to avoid alcohol, however, because it interacts with most antidepressants.

If you agree to take the medication recommended by your general practitioner it could take at least two weeks before you begin to feel better and you may be tempted to stop the treatment before that. Stick with it and there is an excellent chance that you will improve. If your mood does not improve then your general practitioner will change you to another antidepressant. This does not mean your situation is hopeless; in fact a change of drug is necessary in about 30 per cent of people.

Counselling

Understandably, you want to avoid medication and you ask about counselling. There have been several studies comparing counselling with antidepressants in the treatment of depressive illness and the evidence to date suggests that while most people prefer counselling, its effect on symptoms is short lived. However, there is a talking treatment called cognitive therapy that has a better impact on symptoms and your general practitioner may consider referring you for this.

* * *

You can be assured that you will not become addicted to antidepressants, you will not become a zombie and simply changing medication will overcome any serious side effects that you experience. You will also be able to work as normal and can anticipate a positive response.

Useful Reading

McKeon, P. (1997) *Coping with Depression and Elation*, Sheldon Press: London

Useful Website

www.depressiondepot.net

My general practitioner has recently diagnosed depression and started me on antidepressants last week. I don't mind taking them since I know of a lot of people who have been helped by them. However, I wonder how long I will have to take them for and if I will have to stay on them for life. I would hate that. This all began after I moved home having been abroad for several years, so I am hoping that I can avoid stresses such as this and not become ill again.

I am sorry that you have not been feeling well recently but now that you are on the correct treatment you should be feeling much better very soon. It can take a few weeks to notice an improvement, although with some of the latest antidepressants an improvement in mood happens after as little as five to seven days. So you should be feeling somewhat better in the next few days.

Too Early

One of the problems that doctors encounter is that when the person feels well and back to normal, there is a strong temptation to stop medication. This is, of course, entirely understandable but the symptoms can break through very quickly again, especially in the first six months. For this reason, it is recommended that treatment should continue for six to nine months once complete well-being is achieved, although the dose can be reduced during that period.

Recurrence

For many, depression does recur, especially when it is severe and very incapacitating. Among those ill enough to require specialist in-patient treatment, the recurrence rate is about 70 per cent – this is a high figure and although relapse is most likely to occur in the early stages following treatment termination, it can occur at any time after the initial episode, although with a diminishing frequency after the first five years. In order to prevent relapse some are required to take long-term medication and this dramatically improves the prospects of remaining illness free. Some research also suggests that specific talking therapies help in maintaining well-being, although these have to be combined with medication. On their own, talking therapies have not been shown to prevent relapse.

You do not fall into the category described above as you are not severely ill or incapacitated by your illness and are being treated by your general practitioner. These milder illnesses have a much better outlook and the recurrence rate is of the order of 30 per cent, with some studies suggesting that it may be even less than that.

Support

One of the factors associated with a good outcome is having support from loved ones. The importance of having people around you who can offer emotional back-up and practical help when needed has been shown in many recent studies to improve the outcome, even among those with mild depression.

Like you, many people believe that when a depressive illness has a trigger, such as you have experienced, the risk of it recurring must be less. However, this is not correct and it seems that having had a single episode of depression makes one biologically more sensitive to a recurrence, whether or not there was a stressor preceding it. For this reason, you will have an increased risk of depression recurring compared with somebody who never had this illness.

However, as your depression began after you moved back to Ireland it may be that you experienced a type of bereavement for friends that you had to leave or perhaps you were apprehensive at the new life that was ahead of you. You may need to explore this further if you continue to be upset about the move.

* * *

I hope that you will be among the 70–80 per cent who do not have a further episode in the future. However, if you do have a relapse, then you should remember that your illness is treatable and entirely controllable. If you can imagine how high blood pressure can be controlled by medication as well as dietary measures then you might find cause for optimism in the fact that with appropriate treatment your illness can also be controlled. You should not feel stigmatised by having depression and, although it is upsetting, it is not a sign of weakness.

Useful Reading

Salmans, Sandra (1997) *Depression: Questions you Have, Answers you Heed*, Thorsons: London

Useful Contact

AWARE
72 Lower Leeson Street, Dublin 2, Tel. (01) 6617211

Depression and Manic-Depression 75

I was very upset recently to hear about the problems that people experience with the drug "Seroxat". I have been depressed on and off for the last ten years but since starting this antidepressant five years ago, I haven't looked back. I have had none of the problems that others described. However, I am now wondering if I should stop the medication. I am terrified that I may be addicted to it or that I might become suicidal, as was suggested in the media coverage.

It is regrettable that the recent coverage about this drug was so sensational but you have done the right thing in thinking carefully before making any decision about what to do.

SSRIs

The group of antidepressants to which Seroxat belongs are known as the SSRIs and they have been available in this country since the late 1980s. There is a lot of experience with them internationally and they have been found to be very useful in a number of disorders other than depression, including obsessive-compulsive disorder and bulimia nervosa. They can be used in the long term to prevent relapses in depression, which is often a recurring disorder. From what you say in your letter you belong to that category. "Seroxat" is one brand of this medication but its generic name is paroxetine. Its use is not recommended in children but it continues to be licensed for adult use.

Discontinuation

In spite of the fears raised about the possibility of it being addictive, there is no evidence for this at all. In order for any substance to be addictive it must have several features, among them the necessity to increase the dose so as to maintain the effect, known as tolerance, craving, behaviour that is centred around obtaining the substance and physical symptoms on discontinuation. Paroxetine only possesses the last of these features and information about the discontinuation syndrome, as it is called, is provided on the patient information leaflet in the packet. In fact, many medications have discontinuation syndromes associated with them and they are not regarded as addictive. For example, the sudden cessation of steroids can cause major physical complications, and even death, yet this is not due to any addictive property.

Suicide

The other question that has arisen about this drug is the claim that it could cause people to take their own lives by increasing suicidal thoughts. However, depressive illness is an illness that if untreated carries with it a substantial risk of suicide, of the order of 4–7 per cent. It is well recognised among those treating depression that the time of greatest risk for suicide is during the early stages of recovery.

Depressive illness is associated with low motivation, poor concentration and suicidal ideas. Often, before treatment is commenced the person's low level of motivation and poor concentration prevents them from planning or executing any attempt on their life. However, once the antidepressants begin to work, usually within two weeks, concentration and drive improve and this happens before suicidal ideas or hopelessness diminish. It is for this reason that the early stage of treatment is the most dangerous. This danger applies equally with all antidepressants, not just with paroxetine, and it is due to the illness itself rather than its treatment.

* * *

There is a danger that if you stop your medication you will relapse again. You could of course be put on different treatments to prevent recurrence but they may or may not be equally effective for you. I suggest you discuss this with your doctor, but in the absence of any specific problems I would encourage you to be cautious about changing as you have been well for so long.

Useful Reading

McKeon, Patrick and Corcoran, Gillian (1998) *Notes on Depression: Types, Symptoms, Causes and Treatment*, Aware Publications: Dublin

Useful Contact

AWARE
72 Lower Leeson Street, Dublin 2, Tel. (01) 6617211

What is endogenous depression? I was diagnosed with this condition many years ago yet I see very little written about it. How many types of depression are there and are the treatments similar for all?

"Endogenous" depression was the term used to describe a depressive illness that occurred from "within" the person; in other words, there was no external trigger. This was to distinguish it from "reactive" depression, an illness that occurred in response to a stressful event such as loss, job change etc. The typical features of "endogenous" depression were early morning wakening, appetite reduction, constipation, loss of sexual interest and feeling worse in the morning. These were known as the biological features.

Confusing Terminology

However, these terms were dropped in the early 1980s because it became clear that they were confusing. In particular, "reactive" depression was often used inappropriately to describe understandable depression such as that which occurs for many people who have particular worries in their lives, for example marital problems. Depressed mood in these circumstances is now termed a "stress/adjustment reaction" rather than a depressive illness, since it resolves with the passage of time and does not require any special treatment. In addition, it became clear that a depressive illness that had a trigger had the same outcome as "endogenous" depression. In particular, the risk of recurrence was similar in both and after one episode of reactive depression other episodes often followed without a trigger. It is now clear that there is a biological sensitisation of the brain to further episodes once one has occurred. It also became clear that there was considerable overlap between the symptoms in both types.

Modern Descriptions

In current practice we speak of a depressive episode or of recurrent depressive disorder to describe single or repeated episodes, whether or not they have a trigger. These are further divided into those who have accompanying psychotic symptoms, i.e. loss of touch with reality such as hearing voices when there is nobody there, and those who do not. The psychotic type of depression is the most severe, although it is uncommon. In American textbooks, the terms major and minor depression are used to describe these disorders and their different severities.

Dysthymia is another type of depression that is chronic and that often begins at a young age and rumbles on for years. Unlike the other types of depression there are no acute episodes, rather there is the steady presence of distressing symptoms and for this reason it may not even be diagnosed. It can cause huge problems in relationships, as the person is always gloomy and disinterested in activities.

Other Depression

Seasonal affective disorder (SAD) is a type of recurrent depressive disorder that occurs only during the winter months and even without treatment spontaneously resolves as spring approaches.

Post-partum depression is a depressive illness that occurs following childbirth. In some women it is confined exclusively to that time, while in others episodes of depression can occur at any time, whether or not childbirth has occurred.

Manic-depression or bipolar disorder consists of moods that swing violently between depression and mania (over-activity, elation, over-talkativeness).

Treatment

There are some treatment differences although the mainstay of help is with antidepressants. For example, in recurrent depressive disorder, long-term antidepressants may be needed to prevent relapse. In SAD, treatment may only be needed during the risk period and the use of light therapy can also help symptoms to remit. In bipolar disorder, lithium is used to prevent relapse.

Talking treatments may also be used in some of these. For example, cognitive therapy is helpful in depressive episodes, dysthymia and recurrent depression but has not been studied in SAD. Psycho-education about bipolar depression has been found to be helpful in reducing relapse by assisting the person in identifying the signs of early recurrence.

* * *

If you were diagnosed with "endogenous" depression many years ago, you may have the condition that is now called recurrent depressive disorder, but you should ask your doctor for the exact term. You could then get more information from your library or the Internet.

Useful Reading

Salmans, Sandra (1997) *Depression: Questions You Have, Answers You Need*, Thorsons: London

Useful Website

www.psychologynet.org/major.html

Useful Contact

AWARE
72 Lower Leeson Street, Dublin 2, Tel. (01) 6617211

My sister is an in-patient at present and last week was diagnosed as having a mild form of manic-depression. I know very little about this illness and I am worried that she will have to be hospitalised permanently and that she will never get well again. Can you give me any information about this condition?

Manic-depression is an illness in which the person swings from low moods (the depression phase) to being overly excited, talkative and either unnaturally happy or extremely irritable (the manic phase). In recent years the term bipolar disorder is more frequently used in preference to manic-depression, since the older term represents the most serious and obvious form of the illness.

Milder Forms

As your sister has been diagnosed with mild manic-depression, this probably means that she has a form of bipolar disorder known as bipolar 2, in which the "high" phases are barely noticeable. This is to distinguish it from bipolar 1 disorder in which there is gross over-activity and unusual beliefs about having special powers or having a mission, as well as elation and/or irritability. In fact, bipolar 2 is a condition that is often misdiagnosed or even not diagnosed at all, due to the subtle nature of the symptoms.

Treatable

The treatment is the same for both forms of the disorder but it probably does suggest that your sister will be discharged from hospital more quickly. However, she will continue to need medication to prevent relapses and lithium is the drug that is the first choice for this. About 70 per cent of those taking lithium respond very well and do not have further recurrences. If your sister does not respond at all or has only a partial response then other medications are used, including carbamazepine, lamotrigine and sodium valproate (used also for the control of epilepsy). These drugs may also be used in preference to lithium if your sister gets unacceptable side effects such as weight gain or if her moods swing up and down in rapid succession. This form of the disorder is known as rapid cycling bipolar disorder.

Additional Treatments

Some recent studies have found that the addition of cognitive therapy, which is a talking treatment that focuses on the person's immediate coping skills and thought processes, helps prevent relapse, but only in conjunction with a mood-stabilising drug. There is no evidence that talking therapy on its own is helpful. Education about the disorder (psycho-education) has been shown to be helpful in improving the prognosis also, as it helps with acceptance of the illness and its treatment. It also assists in the early identification of relapses.

Positive Future

There is very little doubt but that your sister will be discharged home from hospital and there is a very strong possibility that she can live a normal life, albeit with the inconvenience of having to take medication. She may have to have blood tests every few months also to ensure that she is receiving the correct dose of medication to stay well, but there are many conditions in which blood levels of drugs are used to monitor treatment. I think you can be optimistic about your sister's recovery provided, as with any medical condition, she takes the treatment that is recommended.

* * *

I suggest that with her permission you discuss these matters with her treating doctor and that you encourage her to do the same. I hope she recovers quickly and resumes her old activities as before.

Useful Reading
Jamison, Kay Redfield (1997) *An Unquiet Mind*, Vintage Books: New York

Useful Website
www.pendulum.org

Useful Contact
AWARE
72 Lower Leeson Street, Dublin 2, Tel. (01) 6617211

My best friend is twenty-eight and she has recently been diagnosed as having manic-depression. She has been told she must take lithium but she really doesn't want to, as she fears she may become addicted to it. Can you tell me a bit about this illness and the treatment that has been suggested?

Manic-depression, also called bipolar disorder, is so named because it is associated with bouts of depression when the person becomes gloomy, withdrawn and tearful. The person may also experience an upward swing in mood, often described as a "high" – these are the manic phases of the illness. The "highs" are not just ordinary high spirits; they may be associated with overspending and the normal restraints are replaced by uncharacteristic behaviour such as being crude or sexually provocative. Some people become irritable and get racing thoughts so that their mind feels crowded out. As a result, it may be difficult to follow the train of thought, as varied ideas come flooding in. Often the manic person gets an exaggerated sense of their importance or abilities and is very overactive, needing little sleep and potentially culminating in exhaustion. The overwhelming mood is either one of elation or extreme irritability. Sometimes the highs and lows occur in rapid succession and this is known as rapid cycling disorder. Bipolar disorder affects about 1 per cent of the population and begins in early adulthood, as in your friend's case.

Starting Lithium

The benefits of lithium were first identified in Australia in the 1960s and its discovery revolutionised the treatment of manic-depression. Lithium is a salt that is excreted by the kidneys. For this reason, before starting to take lithium a blood and urine test will have to be done to confirm that kidney function is normal. In a young person such as your friend it is unlikely that there will be any problem of this type. Lithium can affect the thyroid gland so it will be necessary to test this by taking a sample of blood. If lithium does cause the thyroid to under-function or to swell there may be a need to discontinue it, but it is also possible to continue to take it with close monitoring. Finally, an ECG will be required to test heart function.

Monitoring Treatment

One of the benefits of lithium is that the level in the blood at which it is effective is known as a result of the many years of research in its effectiveness. This will require a blood test, done twelve hours after the last dose has been taken, so, for most, this will mean a test in the morning. Initially, the blood level is checked every week but once the required level is reached, three-monthly monitoring is sufficient.

Side Effects

Lithium is not an addictive drug so you can reassure your friend about this. However, she may need to take it for the rest of her life, although some people will wish to have a trial off medication after five years free of relapse. The main side effect is weight gain and this can be upsetting, especially for young women. This results from the effect of lithium on carbohydrate metabolism and from fluid retention and is best managed by healthy eating and exercise. A fine tremor may also develop in some people who take lithium but medication is available to counteract this effect. If the dose of lithium is too high symptoms such as nausea, vomiting and difficulty speaking can occur. For this reason, it will be essential for your friend to have her levels monitored regularly.

If it Does Not Work

Lithium is effective in up to 70 per cent of sufferers. Among those who do not respond, other mood-stabilising agents are used so that, ultimately, for most the disorder is controllable. These can also be used if side effects of lithium are too troublesome. Some medications used to control epilepsy are now used to control bipolar disorder also; in fact in the US, they are more frequently used than lithium. The three drugs most often prescribed instead of lithium or in combination with it are sodium valproate, carbamazepine and lamotrigine. Some are more effective when the predominant mood swing is depression and some when "highs" are more frequent.

Pregnancy

As your friend is young, she may one day wish to have a baby. Early studies of lithium in pregnancy found that up to 10 per cent of babies exposed to this drug in the first three months of pregnancy had congenital abnormalities and for this reason it was recommended that it be discontinued for the first three months of pregnancy. However, recent studies have shown that it is safer than was once thought. Your friend should ask her doctor to obtain information about lithium in pregnancy if she is considering this.

* * *

Your friend can be assured that lithium is an excellent treatment. It does require close monitoring as outlined and provided she does this, her prospects for a normal life are very good indeed.

Useful Reading

Jamison, Kay Redfield (1997) *An Unquiet Mind*, Vintage Books: New York

Useful Website

www.nami.org

Useful Contact

AWARE
72 Lower Leeson Street, Dublin 2, Tel. (01) 6617211

I am fifty and I was in hospital for two weeks. I feel much better now. However, I was surprised when my doctor told me I had depression as I thought I was having a nervous breakdown. I had hoped to go back to work soon (I work in a bank) but if I've had depression then I'm scared to even think about this.

I am delighted you are feeling better again. The phrase "nervous breakdown" is not a medical term but is one used by the public. It means different things to different people: for some it means an acute emotional crisis while for others it can mean a depressive illness, such as you have had. You should not be upset that you have been diagnosed as having depression, since it is a treatable illness in almost everybody.

Returning to Activities

Provided your depression is properly treated and you remain well then there should be no problem about returning to work. You will be the best judge of this and there are no hard and fast guidelines about the time it should take. It is important that you return when you feel able to and that you do not put yourself under any pressure to do so. It is best to delay this until you are first able to cope well in other areas. For example, are you able to manage your family, the shopping and housework? What about social activities – are you able to go out again and meet friends? Since you work in a bank you will have to be confident that your concentration is good so that you won't make mistakes. Also, returning to work will mean that you will be busier than you now are. You will only be able to function in all of these roles if you are sleeping well and waking refreshed. Once you feel that all of these aspects are in order you should approach your boss and work half time for a few weeks until you adjust to the new demands again.

Education

I can understand that you are fearful of going back to work. However, reading about depression will help you understand more about your illness and identify the best approach to coping with it for the future, especially in relation to work and social activities. It will also help you learn about treatments that work and those that do not. For instance, many people think that medication is not necessary and they stop taking it at the first opportunity, when in fact it should be continued for at least six to nine months. Sometimes people think that certain talking therapies are all that is required when in fact those that work are very specific and include cognitive therapy and interpersonal therapy.

Others are not so effective. Reading will also update you on new developments about the causes of depression and the research that is being carried out.

Support Groups

People vary in their attitude to self-help and support groups. I believe they are a good idea provided they work with, rather than against, the medical profession. You should check before you join that they do not oppose medication or try to dissuade people from attending their doctors. Support groups differ from self-help groups in that they do not offer specific help; rather by meeting others with the same condition people feel less isolated. Whichever you choose, you should be mindful that people with different illnesses might also be in the group, as there is no independent check that all the members suffer from the illness for which the group was established.

Stress and Recovery

During the early stages of recovery, such as following discharge from hospital, stress might indeed worsen things. However, once you are taking on your usual responsibilities both at home and at work and are following your doctor's advice, you should be able to deal with stress the same as everybody else. You do not need to be protected any more than anybody else and there is no reason why your life cannot proceed as you had envisaged before your hospitalisation.

* * *

The belief that depression permanently interferes with life is, unfortunately, a common myth.

Useful Reading

Salmans, Sandra (1997) *Depression: Questions You Have, Answers You Need*, Thorsons: London

Useful Website

www.rcpsych.ac.uk
(Click on Mental Health Information and then follow the instructions)

Useful Contacts

AWARE
72 Lower Leeson Street, Dublin 2, Tel. (01) 6617211

Recovery Incorporated
Cherry Orchard, Dublin 10, Tel. (01) 6260775

My husband was depressed a few months ago but he is now feeling much better as a result of his doctor's treatment. We have always had a very good and confiding relationship and his depression, due I think to problems at work, was a great surprise. I am worried that he may be overdoing things and get depressed again. He insists on going back to work and on going out with his friends to play golf again. I don't know how to advise him but I am afraid he is putting too much stress on himself.

It is good news that your husband is well again and he is being perfectly reasonable in wanting to get back to his old routines as soon as possible. Many people fear that too much stress may bring back depression but this is only a problem for a minority of those who suffer with the illness. Your husband should be encouraged to go back to work, provided his symptoms have all resolved and he feels ready to. He might consider returning on a part time-basis for a few weeks, if this option is open to him. He is the best judge of this.

Sleep and Alcohol

The fact that your husband wants to go out socially is also good news and should be encouraged. However, it is important to sound a word of caution. He should guard against late nights, even if this happens only once a week, since a disruption to the normal sleep rhythm could result in a worsening of symptoms or even a full recurrence. It may sound overly cautious but I would suggest that if he reads in bed he should curtail this and turn out the lights by midnight.

The other area of concern is alcohol. There is no suggestion that your husband has a drink problem, but alcohol is a depressant drug and even when consumed in small quantities can worsen depressive symptoms, especially in the early stages of recovery. Many people report feeling terrible, even after two drinks. Alcohol can also interact with some of the drugs used to treat depressive illness causing drowsiness and this is another reason for avoiding alcohol for the time being. Some people are tempted to skip their medication when they are socialising or worry that taking medication too late may be unacceptable. Again missing an antidepressant is inadvisable at this point in his treatment.

Of even greater concern is the tendency of some people to discontinue their treatment because they feel so well. If your husband is on antidepressants, he will need to remain on them for six to nine months and they should be discontinued only under the supervision of his doctor. You can reassure him that this medication is not addictive and that early discontinuation could cause a prompt relapse.

Over-Cautious

Your role now is to remove the protective cloak that you may want to keep around your husband and to encourage him in reintegrating back into everyday life. When he was ill it was important to remove him from some of the responsibilities that he had but you should now regard him as well and treat him as such, bearing in mind the precautions I mentioned earlier. I am sure that if he feels he is overdoing things he will be able to confide in you as he has always done. You can ask him from time to time how he feels but do not overdo it, as he may feel watched and intruded upon. Above all, you must avoid attributing every mood change to his depression but rather try to think back to his habits and behaviours before he was ill – these will not change. Only if there are persisting symptoms or day-to-day problems that are related to depression should you be concerned

* * *

There is a myth that those who have had depression need to be careful to avoid stress and that promotion at work and the usual responsibilities of being a parent, a husband etc. have to be put aside. This is a very inaccurate view and there is no reason why your husband cannot live a totally fulfilling life in every respect.

Useful Reading

Golant, M. and Golant, S.K. (1996) *What to Do when Someone you Love is Depressed*, Henry Holt: New York

Useful Contact

AWARE
72 Lower Leeson Street, Dublin 2, Tel. (01) 6617211

I had a very unhappy childhood. My parents argued a lot and when I was ten they separated. I remained with my mother and we got on very well. In later years, my relationship with my father improved and we now meet every week. I am happily married and my husband is wonderful. I read that unhappiness in childhood such as I experienced causes depression. Is this correct?

This is not correct, but many people assume that it does cause depression. When we speak of something causing an illness we mean that without this factor the illness would not have occurred and its presence is in some way a trigger for this illness.

Risk

It is important to distinguish between a risk factor and a causative factor. The presence of a risk factor implies that the chances of developing the particular illness are increased but it is not inevitable that the illness will occur. For example, being overweight increases the risk of getting high blood pressure but it is not inevitable – other factors come into play in bringing about elevated blood pressure, such as high cholesterol. A risk factor implies that the chances of developing the particular condition are higher in those who possess the risk factor than in those without it.

A large number of risk factors have been identified as associated with depressive illness of which the most pertinent are childhood adversity and trauma, such as loss through divorce or death, especially the former. Since you have experienced this, your risk is increased. Sexual abuse is also an important factor. We often assume that vulnerability is concerned with our past. However, biological factors are also pertinent; in particular, a family history of depressive illness or alcoholism increases the likelihood of becoming depressed but does not make it inevitable. Personality may also be an important risk factor and those who find change difficult would be at risk when faced with a new situation such as moving house or changing job. The single biggest risk for developing depression is having had a previous episode.

Causation

A causative factor is the trigger for a particular illness and for depression this can be bereavement and other loss events. Sometimes the event may be pleasant as with post-natal depression, which is triggered by childbirth, even when there is much joy at the pregnancy and birth. Other triggers include moving house, being involved in an accident or changing to a new job. Physical illness, especially one that is painful, may lead to a depressive illness and some medications may also induce depression. However, since not everybody experiencing a bereavement or giving birth will develop a clinical depression it is clear that the background risk factors described above must also be present.

Protection

Even when an individual possesses a vulnerability factor, such as you possess, and experiences a stressful event that might be a trigger, they may be protected from depression by having confidants, as you seem to have in your husband. Being able to access practical help when there are difficulties is also beneficial. Some studies show that having religious beliefs is a protection. Moreover, those who deal with events by confronting them rather than by avoiding them reduce their risk also.

Interaction

So it is really the interplay between personal vulnerability, whether environmental or biological, the occurrence of stressful events and the presence of protective factors that leads to clinical depression. At particular risk are those who have had a previous depressive episode. However, a large number, probably up to 30 per cent, have no stressful event triggering the illness and in this group the biological vulnerability is very high, resulting in spontaneous depression or what used to be called endogenous depression.

* * *

It is clear that the mixture of risk and triggering factors that culminate in clinical depression is complex and there is no definitive way of proving that an individual will become depressed in later life, as protective factors also play a part. It is an over-simplification for you to assume that because of childhood problems with your parent you will inevitably become depressed, since you now have protection in a good marriage.

Useful Reading

Jamison, Kay Redfield (1997) *An Unquiet Mind*, Vintage Books: New York

Useful Website

www. allaboutdepression.com

Useful Contact

AWARE

72 Lower Leeson Street, Dublin 2, Tel. (01) 6617211

I have recently been diagnosed with depression and am receiving treatment from my doctor. I am delighted that I am getting better but I am worried that I will pass it on to my children. I have two children and I would love to have another but I hate to think of them becoming ill like me. Can you tell me what is the risk of them inheriting it?

I am glad that you are getting better. Many people do not seem to realise that depression is a treatable illness provided it is correctly diagnosed and that treatment is complied with, which can be a problem for many, who see it as a weakness to be fought against.

Genetic Basis

It is true that in some people there is a genetic component to their depression, especially manic-depression, known also as bipolar disorder. For example, if one parent has bipolar disorder the children have an eight to eighteen times chance of developing the same condition. However, for those with depression only, also called unipolar disorder, the risk is about two to three times higher when compared to the children of those without depression. From these figures it is clear that there is no certainty of inheriting the disorder. Social and environmental factors, such as personal supports and adverse stressful events, also play a large part, especially in bringing about the first episode.

Family and Adoption Studies

Family studies suggest that those with depressive illness are about twice as likely to have a close relative with the same condition as compared to non-depressed controls. This has also been confirmed by two of three recent well-designed adoption studies in which the adopted children of depressed parents were followed through to adulthood and showed a somewhat increased risk of developing depressive illness in later life. Similarly, studies of twins suggest that there is a genetic component to depression. Identical twins have an increased risk, known as concordance, of about 50 per cent, where one already has the disorder. The concordance among non-identical twins is much lower, ranging between 5 and 25 per cent, depending on the study.

Which Gene?

Some recent work has tried to identify which gene is implicated. However, results are contradictory with some suggesting chromosome 5, some chromosome 11 and others describing an association with the same gene that causes colour blindness. So there is no certainty with regard to the responsible gene or genes. In all probability there are likely to be several genes involved rather than a single, specific gene.

You should remember, however, that it is not the illness *per se* which is inherited but an increased risk or vulnerability to developing it under certain circumstances. In view of the multiple risk factors and causes of depressive illness and the complexity of the genetic inheritance, there is no ball-park figure that can be offered in relation to the risk of your children becoming depressed at some stage later in life.

Post-Natal Depression

Recent studies suggest a greater risk of passing on depression comes from the impact that the illness has on the early mother-child interaction rather than from the gene pool. A mother with clinical depression that is untreated will have difficulty nurturing the young child and this in turn may impact upon the child's developing personality. This means that obtaining prompt and adequate treatment is essential if you are depressed in the future and have a young child.

* * *

In summary, there is no certainty that you have passed on depressive illness to your children, since a genetic predisposition is just one of many factors that is associated with it. I suggest that you discuss this with your doctor who may refer you to a specialist so that you can get more detailed information.

Useful Reading

Salmons, Sandra (1997) *Depression: Questions you Have, Answers you Need*, Thorsons: London

Useful Website

www.psycom.net/depression.central.genetics.html

I am thirty-two and had my first a baby six weeks ago. Since she arrived I have been feeling tearful and sad. I thought it was the "baby blues" but now I think it must be more as it has gone on so long. I feel so guilty because I should be happy. I find every day a struggle and my husband has to help me cope with her. My general practitioner says I have post-natal depression and he has prescribed antidepressants. I had planned to have another baby but now I'm not so sure, as I am afraid that I would get depressed again. What should I do?

I am sure you must be very surprised that you feel so low after such a happy event but post-natal depression is common – up to 10 per cent of women develop this condition in the months following childbirth. Your general practitioner was correct to prescribe antidepressants as they are a very effective treatment and you should feel better within a few weeks of starting them.

Support

A further aspect to your treatment is the availability of people to support you during this period, which will probably only last a few weeks. You should ask family members, friends or in-laws to give you some help with the baby, the housework etc. in the short term. Isolation is known to be one of the factors delaying recovery from this illness. Night-time help would also be beneficial so as to allow you get a full nights' sleep, although I know this may be difficult to organise, especially if your husband is working. Perhaps you could get help even one night each week for the next month or so.

Subsequent Pregnancies

Your fear that you may become depressed if you have other babies is understandable. Research suggests that those with post-natal depression are divided into two broad groups: those who get depressed only in association with pregnancy and those who get depressed at other times also. The first group may initially show symptoms during pregnancy with a worsening after delivery. The second and more common category usually has no problems during pregnancy but after delivery show the symptoms of depressive illness and can subsequently develop symptoms after other stressful events such as moving house, bereavement and so on, or indeed without any stressor.

Prevention

It is recommended that those at risk of a recurrence of post-natal depression following subsequent pregnancies be given preventative antidepressants, commencing the day following delivery and continuing for about three months. This approach is particularly important when the depression is very severe and incapacitating. If the illness is not so incapacitating some women chose to avoid medication until (and if) the illness emerges in subsequent weeks. In these circumstances, treatment with antidepressants is for about six months.

Accepting Treatment

The most important aspect of your problem now and for the future is that you seek and accept treatment, as there is a lot of research data showing that very young children whose mothers are clinically depressed are at risk themselves of future depression, not due to transmission of the illness through genes but as a result of the impaired relationship during the early months of the child's life.

* * *

Even in the worst-case scenario with an illness developing following a subsequent pregnancy, this is a very treatable illness. You do not necessarily need to limit your family to one on the basis of having had post-natal depression. There are several specialists in peri-natal psychiatry in Ireland and your general practitioner will advise you on whether you should consult one regarding the risks associated with future pregnancies and preventing further episodes of post-natal depression.

Useful Reading

Corry, Dr Martina (1991) *Post-Natal Depression: A Guide for Mothers and Families*, Available from AWARE, Tel. (01) 6617211

Useful Websites

www.chss.iup.edu/postpartum

http://www.rcpsych.ac.uk/info/help/depintro/
(Click on post-natal depression)

I have suffered with post-natal depression in the past and my doctor says I should take antidepressants for a few months after delivery to prevent it recurring following this pregnancy. I am scared, as I want to breast-feed my baby.

Congratulations and good luck with your new baby. Your doctor is correct. It is considered best to prevent post-natal depression recurring in those who have had it in the past by prescribing antidepressants for about three months beginning just before delivery. Like you, many mothers are fearful of this approach, since they worry that these drugs will be excreted in breast milk. However, there is now a lot of information available on the safety of breastfeeding in these circumstances and it is positive. Most women take antidepressants when breastfeeding without any reported problems for the baby and with the added advantage of being able to enjoy the early weeks with the baby free from the burden of depression.

Older Antidepressants

In general, the older antidepressants are recommended to breastfeeding mothers because there is most information available on them, gathered over forty years of their use. Drugs in this group of antidepressants, known as the tricyclic group, are excreted in tiny amounts in breast milk, so that an adverse effect on the newborn baby is highly unlikely. However, it is recommended that if any excessive drowsiness is noticed then this should be drawn to the attention of the treating doctor.

Newer Antidepressants

The antidepressants that came on the market in the late 1980s, known as the SSRI group, of which "prozac" is the best known, are considered to be safe in these circumstances also. The very new groups, available for the past five years or less, may be safe, but as they will not yet have stood the test of time or been monitored in large numbers of patients they are best taken with caution. In other words, there is too little information available to say, one way or the other, if they are safe. However, much depends on the medication you had previously and if you encountered no problems then consideration should be given to this again.

Avoiding Antidepressants

Many women opt to avoid all medication and to take a chance that they will not get depressed. This is certainly a possibility, especially if you have had pregnancies after which you did not develop depression. However, if you have been depressed after several pregnancies there is a strong possibility that this will happen again. Your history can be a rough guide to what may happen after this pregnancy.

Most mothers do not realise that having an untreated post-natal depression may have a negative effect on the baby, so this is an important consideration. In fact, the impact of depression on the baby is probably worse than not breastfeeding. This could be a win-win situation for you if you can both prevent depression and feed your baby yourself.

Information

Every packet of tablets now, by law, contains a patient information leaflet in which data on the safety of medication in a variety of circumstances is discussed. Your doctor could also write to the manufacturers for information that they have from trials of the drug and from patient monitoring. Following the release of a drug onto the market, all companies are by law compelled to carry out a surveillance for unwanted effects that develop in those for whom the treatment is prescribed and the results of this can be made available. Finally, the Internet is a rich source of information and I have provided a very good website address as well as the name of a booklet that you may find helpful in reaching a decision.

*　*　*

This is an important decision for you and especially for your baby.

Useful Reading

Corry, Dr Martina (1999) *Post-Natal Depression: A Guide for Mothers and Families*, available from AWARE, Tel. (01) 6617211

Useful Website

www.depression.about.com
(Go to portal on female depression)

I am twenty-eight and I now hate the winter because I become gloomy and unhappy at this time every year. I find each day a struggle. I usually try to get away for a winter sun holiday, which helps a lot. My husband says everybody feels low during the winter months but I don't know of many people for whom it's a real struggle. Could I have SAD and what can I do about it?

Seasonal affective disorder (SAD) is the term used to describe a group of symptoms that occur annually between September and March, very similar to those that you describe. So you could indeed have this disorder.

Both Hemispheres

This condition occurs mainly in women, who comprise 80 per cent of sufferers. Like you, most are in the under-forty age bracket and the usual age at which the symptoms first become apparent is between eighteen and thirty. This condition is found among those living in both hemispheres, but is almost unknown among those who live within 30 degrees north or south of the equator. Light, therefore, seems to be a crucial element in its causation, although it is not the only important factor, since there is frequently a family history of depressive illness or of alcoholism.

Craving for Sleep and Food

The main features of SAD are excessive lethargy such as you describe, which may lead to difficulties going to work or going out socially. In addition, there is often a craving for sleep and for carbohydrates, such as chocolate, during this period. Mood is very low and there may be tearfulness. In spite of the food craving, appetite is otherwise decreased and there may be weight loss.

One of the reasons that many people do not seek professional help is that the symptoms are thought to be understandable in the circumstances. Another reason may lie in the fact that they resolve spontaneously in March or April. Indeed, following their resolution there may be a brief period of over-activity or elation with reduced sleep.

Light Therapy

As you describe, this can be a very incapacitating condition but help is available. Many people request a trial of light therapy. In 1984, the first experiment using light therapy found that it relieved symptoms in a proportion of sufferers.

However, the amount of time for which one must sit beside light varies from individual to individual, averaging about one to two hours. If you have a job that would allow you facility then you may want to try it. The wattage of the light is ten times higher than the usual light bulb and sunglasses must not be worn (it is safe to look into the light). A special light box must be purchased from a medical supplier. However, before you embark upon this treatment you must consult your doctor, who may refer you to a psychiatrist.

Self-Help

You are doing the correct thing in going to winter sun. If possible you should also schedule activities by day, so as to coincide with any sunlight that is available. Exercise is also helpful as it boosts melatonin, the hormone thought to be involved in SAD. If you work in an office that does not have any natural light you may also be vulnerable to this disorder and your working environment should be explored with your employer.

* * *

If light and exercise fail, antidepressant medication, commencing as the symptoms begin and discontinuing in March, may be required. Above all, do not despair. This is a treatable condition and you must seek professional assistance now.

Useful Website

www.nosad.org

Eating Disorders

Every man should eat and drink and enjoy the good of all his labour. It is the gift of God.

Bible, Ecclesiastes, 3:13

My sixteen-year old daughter has recently begun to diet and she has lost two stone in two months. She is "skin and bone" (she never was fat). She said she hated the shape of her body and went on a drastic diet with one of her friends. She has become a very sad girl and our relationship has deteriorated so much because we argue about food all the time. I am scared that she has anorexia nervosa yet I don't believe I should force her to a doctor, as I fear that she will have to go to hospital. I think I could persuade her to see a counsellor though. What do you think?

The history that you give to me unfortunately suggests that your daughter has anorexia nervosa. There may be other tell-tale signs, such as vomiting, hiding food, exercising or taking laxatives. Perhaps her periods have stopped or become irregular. Occasionally those with anorexia nervosa hoard or steal food even though they do not eat it.

Parents Upset

It is certainly very upsetting for parents when their children start to diet excessively and it does not surprise me that you and she are arguing. As the young person's weight drops the sense of being fat increases and with it the need to diet.

Difficult though it may be for you, you should if possible avoid any discussion about food and try to talk with her about other things, since anorexia nervosa is a condition not so much about weight as about other problems. If she can be encouraged to confide in you about these other worries she would have made a start in overcoming her anorexia.

Professional Help

You should certainly take your daughter to a doctor, as anorexia nervosa can lead to very serious physical problems. Also, if she finds it difficult to confide in you she may feel able to open up to a professional. Depending on her physical condition and the amount of weight loss, a period in hospital may be required. If her weight drops to the extent that her long-term health is at risk then she will almost certainly have to be admitted to a medical ward for investigations and weight gain.

It would be a positive move if she did see a "counsellor", but first her physical condition must be evaluated. Your general practitioner will be able to advise you on the appropriate professional to consult. You must also be cautious and refrain from choosing somebody yourself, since this is a complicated and difficult disorder to treat and only a clinical psychologist, behaviour therapist or psychiatrist with specialist knowledge of this condition should be considered. Non-directive counselling would be inappropriate. The preferred treatments are psychodynamic or cognitive therapy. Competence in these therapies is therefore essential.

Therapeutic Relationship

The therapist will be unlikely to try to "persuade" your daughter to start eating and this may perplex you in the beginning. The reason for this is that it would prevent a positive relationship developing between her and the therapist. It would also distract from the underlying difficulties your daughter is experiencing, of which her eating habit is a symptom, and it would appear to her that her fears are being misunderstood.

Sometimes family therapy is required to bring about change in the approach and attitude of the family to the problem but it will be for the therapist to decide if it is required in this instance. Medication does not improve the core symptoms but when depression supervenes, as it often does, it may require treatment of itself. This should not interfere with the ongoing psychotherapy in any way.

* * *

Treatment is lengthy and unfortunately there are no quick solutions. Time and again your daughter may sabotage treatment, but with persistence and effort things can dramatically improve.

Useful Websites

www.grohol.com/disorders

www.rcpsych.ac.uk
(Click on Mental Health Information and then go to appropriate drop-down panel for anorexia)

Useful Contact

Eating Disorder Association of Ireland
Central Office PO Box 8114, Dublin 6, Tel. (01) 4126690

I am twenty-two and have bulimia nervosa. I am terrified of Christmas as I know I will eat myself to the point of sickness. Then I will feel even more guilty than before. I know also that my family will find it difficult and will be on edge all the time, wondering if I'm stuffing myself with food or in the toilet vomiting. I hate being like this and I hate myself for doing this to my family.

Christmas is certainly a very difficult time for many people, including those who are bereaved, lonely, ill or, like you, those who have eating disorders. I understand that you are fearful of overeating at Christmas, since it is a time when there is permission to gorge. Many people find the excesses of Christmas difficult to cope with. However, if you want to remove yourself from the temptation presented by the festivities you might consider some voluntary work on Christmas day so that you are not face to face with the extravagance of Christmas food. Helping in a hostel for the homeless is one way of doing this. Of course, you may feel that you want to be with your family and if you do remain with them there are some simple steps that can be taken to reduce your problem.

Relax

One of the difficulties that many people with eating disorders have is that they are very tense around food and cannot "let go" of their thoughts and anxieties around it. However, you should allow yourself to forget about food and about your problem just for the few days of Christmas. Try doing things that you enjoy and that help you feel contented. If you continue to worry about food, you will find it very difficult to achieve that. Why not play relaxing music and tapes, the kind you enjoyed before your eating disorder started? Activities such as walking or cycling can be very satisfying and can also act as a distraction when you are tempted to think about food. The recurring thoughts about food can also be diverted by simple things such as getting a video that really engages you or by doing yoga and other relaxation exercises.

Family

You will probably feel under surveillance by your parents, especially when you are out of sight, as they will worry that you may be in the kitchen or the bathroom. Why not speak with them and ask them to curtail the spread of food and tell them that in turn you will do all in your power to distract yourself from eating. If you do binge I suggest that you do not discuss this with them over the holiday period, as it will refocus the whole family on food, something you must avoid.

If your family is visiting relatives or friends over the holiday period you should be the one to decide whether to visit with them or not. Resisting food can be very difficult when it is being forced upon you out of Christmas generosity. Rather than going along passively you should explain your predicament to your parents if this arises.

Reward

You may find it helpful to break down your day into four-hour chunks – in that way the holiday period will not be so daunting. You can allocate some pleasurable and distracting activity to each slot and each one that is free from bingeing and vomiting should be awarded a point, leading to a reward if a specific threshold is reached by the end of seven days.

***

When Christmas is over, you should seek professional help to address your eating difficulty.

Useful Websites

www.rcpsych.ac.uk
(Click on Mental Health Information and then go to appropriate drop-down panel for bulimia)

www.grohol.com/disorders

Useful Contact

Eating Disorder Association of Ireland
Central Office PO Box 8114, Dublin 6, Tel. (01) 4126690

Insomnia

Oh sleep! It is a gentle thing
Beloved from pole to pole

Samuel Taylor Coleridge,
The Rime of the Ancient Mariner

Insomnia

I have had trouble sleeping for a number of years. I have tried everything from exercising, to herbal remedies, to tablets, yet I cannot get off to sleep or I wake several times during the night. I never feel refreshed and this causes me problems at work from time to time as I am constantly exhausted, my concentration is badly affected and I'm irritable. Is there anything else I can do?

It is important to bear in mind that some people need less sleep than others. For example Mrs Thatcher was renowned for only requiring five hours each night. You probably do not fit into this category as your performance at work does seem to be impaired. Also, as people get older less sleep is required so your insomnia may be age related, although this change does not usually manifest itself until past sixty-five and you may be younger than this.

Finding a Cause

The first thing is to rule out any causes of insomnia that are related to physical illness such as pain from any condition or shortness of breath due to heart disease or asthma. The second consideration is to rule out psychological conditions such as depressive illness or an anxiety disorder. Both of these are associated with difficulty initiating sleep and in addition depressive illness can cause early wakening after which there is an inability to get back to sleep again. Even though your insomnia is of long standing both of these conditions can also be prolonged unless recognised and treated. If you have either a depressive illness or an anxiety disorder, even in mild form, you would have other symptoms also such as tearfulness, poor concentration and feelings of tension and worry for no reason. Your doctor will tell you if you have any of the array of physical or psychological illnesses associated with insomnia.

Lifestyle – Thou Shalt Not …

If the common physical and psychological causes have been ruled out by your doctor you need to consider lifestyle habits that may be contributing to your insomnia. Alcohol has very dramatic effects on sleep. Many insomnia sufferers take a drink before going to bed because of its initial effect in inducing sleep. However, as the night progresses alcohol causes periods of insomnia. If you drink very regularly you should consider cutting it out for a period of several weeks. This is in no way to suggest that you may have a drink problem but to recommend that you monitor the impact this has on your sleep pattern.

Similarly, beverages containing caffeine such as tea and coffee should be eliminated, or, if you must have them, take them early in the day and use decaffeinated coffee. Nicotine is also a stimulant and so you should not smoke before going to bed. You should also avoid eating heavy meals late at night.

Perhaps you are so tired in the evenings that you nap when you come home from work. This is not a good idea nor is staying in bed at weekends when you feel tired. Only spend as much time in bed on any day as you did prior to the occurrence of this problem.

Lifestyle – Thou Shall ...

Exercise is helpful in the management of sleeplessness but should only be done early in the day as it can act as a stimulant. This is important to remember as the days get longer and we are tempted to make the most of them with evening walks. A warm (not hot) bath lasting about twenty minutes an hour or so before bed-time can be relaxing as can relaxation techniques such as meditation, praying and progressive muscle relaxation – as well as boring activities such as counting sheep! You should replace television viewing before bed with either light reading or gentle radio listening. There are wonderful recordings (available on tape or CD) of running streams and bird-song that are especially soothing.

Changing to another room might be helpful and if you are not asleep within five minutes of going to bed you should get up and do something else – this will help break the connection between bed and not sleeping and will also eliminate the fear of disturbing your partner, itself often a cause of tension. Maintain comfortable sleeping conditions – people vary in their preference for mattress type, keeping the windows open or closed etc. If your insomnia is related to work and fear of forgetting tasks then keep a note pad beside your bed for your reminders. You may have laughed at your granny taking a hot milky drink to bed, but research has shown that it is a very useful hypnotic, as good as medication.

Medication

If these lifestyle suggestions fail then medication may have a part to play, used either episodically or continuously, especially some of the newer preparations that are not associated with the need to increase the dose over time. Some people understandably wish to avoid medication for what should be a normal bodily function but this must be balanced against the effects that insomnia is having on you and your life.

Your doctor might also consider referring you for sleep studies. These are non-painful, non-invasive investigations that would rule out specific sleep disorders such as sleep apnoea. Although uncommon, these disorders are usually treatable.

* * *

I hope you start sleeping better and that your quality of life then improves significantly.

Useful Websites

www.plsgroup.com/insomnia.htm

www.emedicine.com
(Click on sleep disorder centre)

I am constantly tired and exhausted but I cannot sleep at night. I have been to my doctor and he thinks it may be depression. This surprises me because I have nothing to be depressed about. In fact, I don't feel low in mood at all, although I am a bit more emotional than usual. However, I think this is because of my age and my children leaving home.

I am glad that you have been to see your doctor. I presume that he did some blood tests to make sure you did not have anaemia or any physical problem to explain your tiredness. Are you in pain or discomfort and not able to sleep because of that? Assuming that there is no obvious physical explanation then your doctor is quite right to keep depression in mind as a possible cause.

Masked Depression

Surprisingly, it is possible to be depressed without having the typical symptoms. There is a condition, not often talked about in textbooks of mental health nowadays, but one that is clearly recognised, called "masked depression". With masked depression, the depressed mood is hidden but other symptoms manifest it: in the same way that not everybody with a heart attack gets chest pain – there are other manifestations such as pain in the arm or even stomach pain – some people present with symptoms of anxiety, difficulty swallowing, loss of appetite, weight loss or insomnia. It is therefore possible that you may have this form of depression.

Symptoms

Insomnia, without any obvious cause, is very common in depression although less frequently there may be excessive sleeping, known as hypersomnia. The pattern of insomnia is often one of getting off to sleep easily but waking several hours earlier than usual in the morning and not being able to sleep again. Sometimes the person may lie awake for hours, worrying about trivial matters but unable to put them out of their mind, eventually getting to sleep many hours later. Least common is the pattern of waking on and off during the night. Whichever pattern is described, it is inevitably accompanied by tiredness and exhaustion during the day, such as you describe, and the person may even drop off to sleep briefly during the day. Even those who do manage to get eight hours broken sleep say that their sleep is not refreshing.

Coping with Insomnia

You may find it might beneficial to carry out the simple sleep hygiene measures suggested in the previous question, such as getting up at the same time every morning, avoiding caffeine or alcohol at night and ensuring that you are in a relaxed state before getting into bed. In the short term your doctor might prescribe a sleeping tablet. A good night's sleep will certainly make you feel much better. However, the effect may be short lived and other symptoms could break through unless you have treatment for the possible depression. Also, some sleeping tablets can cause dependence, so they should not be taken for more than a few weeks.

* * *

Ultimately, you will need to be properly treated for whatever is causing your symptoms and if it is depression that will mean taking antidepressants. Once you begin to respond your sleep will improve dramatically.

Useful Reading

Ball, Nigel and Hough, Nick (1999) *The Sleep Solution*, Ulysses Press: Berkeley CA

Nicol, Rosemary (1993) *Sleep like a Dream the Drug-Free Way*, Sheldon Press: London

Useful Website

www.nhlbi.nih.gov
(Search for "Facts about insomnia")

Medico-Legal

Morality cannot be legislated but behaviour can be regulated. Judicial decrees may not change the heart but they can restrain the heartless.

Martin Luther King,
Strength of Love, *1963*

I am thirty-two and have been married for two years. There have been problems from the beginning and my husband is now seeking an annulment from the State and from the Church. He says that I am mad and should never have married. I am very upset because I did have a brief admission to a psychiatric unit four years ago – I had trouble coming to terms with my mother's death but I was only there for four days. I did definitely love my husband and was thrilled to marry him. Can he do this?

A marriage annulment means that your marriage would be regarded as never having been valid and therefore any legal or financial responsibility to you might also be forfeited. Your husband is perfectly entitled to seek to annul your marriage, although this does not mean that he will succeed. Many people still opt for annulment rather than divorce when there is a strong feeling that the marriage never really existed.

Grounds

In the past the most common ground for seeking and obtaining an annulment was failure to consummate the marriage due to a physical or psychological problem in either partner. So in men impotence due to medical conditions such as diabetes mellitus or neurological diseases was considered a possible reason and in women failure to consummate due to vaginismus would have been considered.

Other grounds for considering annulment are the ability to give full and free consent to the marriage. This means that each spouse must have freely agreed to the marriage and been free from any outside pressure. If undue pressure came from parents, say because of a pregnancy, then that marriage might be invalid. Similarly, if at the time of marrying the person had a psychiatric problem so that there was not a full understanding of the responsibilities of marriage this might also make it invalid. This might include acute psychiatric illness such as schizophrenia or severe depression. However, if the spouse was well at the time of marriage and only had a past history of any of these conditions such as you outline in your case the validity of the marriage is very unlikely to be affected.

Personality Factors

In the 1980s and 1990s, the thinking in relation to annulment further shifted and personality factors began to be taken into account also, so that those people who were severely immature or irresponsible in their relationships at the time of marriage were also considered in some cases as unable to understand or undertake the responsibilities of marriage. This amounted to considering what is known as personality disorder as grounds for annulment. This of course does not mean that everybody with such a condition has an invalid marriage, since any relationship depends on the interaction between the couple. For example, a marriage between a very dependent person and a very controlling spouse might work well with each meeting the needs of the other; but if two very controlling people married major problems might ensue as each tries to dominate the other. Each application for annulment has to be considered on its own merits, since there is no blanket rule.

Legal Advice

At this point you need legal advice. For the State annulment you will probably be requested by your husband's team to see a psychiatrist representing him for an independent evaluation. Your team will in turn ask your doctors to provide a report of your psychological sate at the time of your marriage and whether this could have interfered with your understanding of marriage or your ability to give consent. The case will be heard in court and in camera so the public will have no knowledge of this. For the Church annulment a representative from the Diocesan Marriage Tribunal will interview you, as well as your husband. You will also be asked to nominate somebody who can provide objective information about you as a person – this might be a close friend or family member.

* * *

Obtaining either a State or Church annulment is a long process and there is no guarantee that your husband will succeed.

Useful Contact

Diocesan Marriage Tribunal
Dublin Office Tel. (01) 8379253

Medico-Legal

I have been advised by my solicitor to see a psychiatrist following a road traffic accident I was involved in. I have become very upset, thinking about it all the time, and I feel I may be depressed. I was depressed following the break-up of my marriage several years ago but I have been well until the recent event. I am terrified that the psychiatrist's report will mention the previous depression, as I told nobody about it. Should I ask the psychiatrist to omit it?

I am sorry to hear about your accident and that you are feeling unwell. You should begin by going to see your general practitioner, who may be able to treat you without referring you to a psychiatrist. In fact, general practitioners treat most of those with emotional disturbances without having to refer them to the specialist services. However, if your doctor feels you need to see a specialist then this can be arranged. It is definitely not a good idea for your solicitor to refer you to a specialist as this may be misconstrued as trying to construct a case for the court rather than being a medical necessity.

Court Report

Your general practitioner can provide a report if necessary and if you do see a psychiatrist then they will also be asked for a report outlining your illness, its link, if any, to the accident and the treatment and likely outcome of your condition. There is a very strong possibility that the report will have to mention your previous depressive episode, since it is probably relevant to your present difficulties. Once a person has had an episode of depression, as you have had, then there is a risk of recurrence in the future and this is true whether there was a life stress causing it or not.

The psychiatrist may conclude that by virtue of having had a prior depression you were at risk for further episodes and that the accident was the trigger in this instance. This is not to suggest that the accident was not important in bringing about this relapse, it merely clarifies that you had a prior vulnerability. This is known as the "egg-shell" principle in legal practice.

Truthfulness

On no account must you ask your doctor or psychiatrist to omit material from the report, since anything that is relevant to your problems now must be incorporated. This would appear as an unwarranted attempt to interfere with a professional witness and certainly would not look good for you. Moreover, failing to include relevant information about previous illnesses could mislead those considering the merits of your case. It would also mean that your legal team would not have all the information relevant to you available to them. Likewise, you should not be tempted to withhold information from your doctor – it is essential that you be open and truthful, even if it is sensitive.

Non-Biased

There is an obligation on professionals working on medico-legal cases to be always non-biased and objective. This means that if a doctor considers that an accident did not cause a particular problem it must be stated in the report even though the patient may disagree. Many people fail to understand this and think that their medical experts will always be on their side and support their claim. Doctors, like any other professionals, are not "hired guns" and so your doctor must provide a report written with a sense of fairness and integrity. Your solicitor will then advise you on whether it will be used in your case.

As well as seeing your own doctor, the insurance company will require you to attend a doctor of their choosing for an independent evaluation, and this doctor too must be impartial and provide an honest report. Both sets of doctors then usually consult with each other in order to identify areas of agreement and disagreement.

* * *

If your previous depression is so sensitive to you, you may decide against pursuing your case for psychological damage. You can discuss this with your solicitor but ultimately you will be the person to make the decision. You must always presume that your case will go to court and that all the information in the reports could get into the public domain.

Taking an action for damages is lengthy and stressful and sometimes can prolong the symptoms, not least because of having to repeat the history over and over to the health professionals that you will have to see. You must think carefully before you proceed and I hope you make the right decision.

Useful Contact

The Law Society
Blackhall Place, Dublin 7, Tel. (01) 6724800

I have suffered with depression for several years but I have never been admitted to hospital for it. In fact, I was last depressed six years ago, just after my last baby was born. I was referred to a very helpful psychiatrist at that time and I haven't looked back since. Unfortunately, my marriage has broken up and my husband now says he will fight for custody of our three children as he maintains that I am unfit to care for them, due to my depression. I am terribly worried that a court will believe him and not me even though he has never expressed any concern about this before.

Unfortunately, court disputes between couples who separate commonly involve children. It is important that what is best for the children is considered and that their welfare and happiness are not sacrificed during the custody battle.

Independent Assessment

You may find comfort from the fact that in making decisions about the custody of your children the judge will have access to a lot of material from your general practitioner, from your psychiatrist and also from an independent child psychiatrist or social worker with expertise in this area whom the court will appoint to interview both you and your husband. This person will visit you at home; they will also visit your husband in his home. In fact, it may be necessary, and usually is, to make several visits in order to make a thorough assessment of the situation.

Children Interviewed

The purpose of this is to decide what is the best arrangement or set of arrangements for all of your children rather than to establish what you or your husband view as the ideal result. If your children are old enough they may be interviewed and if they are teenagers they may have some input into the final decision. The psychiatrist may also meet your children's grandparents if necessary, in order to be satisfied that the children are not being damaged emotionally or in any other respect by either of the parties involved.

Very occasionally, the judge may even meet the children himself in order to be satisfied that they are conversant with what is at stake, although this would only be likely to happen if they were teenagers. In making a decision the judge will not be just relying on word of mouth from you or your husband but on material from a number of professionals, including those who have known you over a number of years.

Depression

Depression is a common condition and in reality is no barrier to being a good parent or to being given custody, either singly or jointly with your husband. It is unclear how well you coped when you were depressed: many people even when depressed and struggling in other areas of their lives are still able to parent children and show them the love and care that they require. If, however, you have a history of being aggressive to your children when depressed or of drinking when ill, that will be taken into consideration. That you appear to have complied with your treatment, are now well and have not been ill for several years will be taken into account also.

Going to Court

It would be misleading if I pretended that going to court to resolve a custody dispute is ever easy. On the contrary, the whole hearing can be fraught with claim and counter claim being made by each party. You may need a little extra support from your general practitioner or psychiatrist over the coming months. You must instruct a solicitor who is knowledgeable about family law (nowadays most solicitors do a lot of family work). If you cannot afford to pay you are entitled to free legal aid. The psychiatrist who treated you will probably be asked to prepare a report and possibly to give evidence and you should ask your solicitor to show you the report that they provide concerning your illness.

* * *

All in all, the fact that you have been well for a number of years, your ability to parent has never been an issue until recently and you are continuing to comply with treatment points to a positive outcome for you.

Useful Contact

Legal Aid Board
Montague Court, 7–11 Montague Street, Dublin 2
Tel. 1899 990 61 52 00

Medico-Legal

My husband and I do not get on. We have been married for twenty-five years and our children are all away from home. He tells me that I am impossible to live with and that I must be psychiatrically unwell. This is totally untrue. I have never had any emotional problems in my life and my general practitioner can confirm this. In fact, when I discussed it with her recently she assured me that I was fine and that I must be a very strong person to put up with my husband's demands. However, I am terrified, as my husband has recently started threatening to have me committed to a psychiatric hospital. Can he do this?

You can be assured that your husband cannot do this. People can sometimes be admitted for psychiatric assessment and/or treatment against their will but evidence of possible serious acute emotional disturbance must be demonstrated. The usual grounds for compulsory admission are the protection of the patient or of others from the consequences of severe mental illness. The law on this dates to 1945; new legislation has been drafted but has not yet come into effect.

Safety of Self or Others

Probably the most common reason for certification is when the person is thought to be suicidal and is refusing treatment. If a person is so severely depressed that life or health is at risk from suicide, starvation or agitation then compulsory admission may be necessary. Sometimes due to severe psychiatric illness behaviour is unpredictable and if the safety of others is threatened then certification for assessment and treatment may be required.

Occasionally, when a person is behaving violently compulsory admission is suggested. However, in the absence of possible mental illness as a cause this would also be illegal. So having a violent personality is not a ground for certification.

A person with alcohol abuse cannot be admitted against their will unless of course they are suicidal or severely depressed. Arguments between spouses or relatives due to relationship problems, such as you mention with your husband, are not grounds for compulsory admission.

Process

To apply for compulsory admission the next of kin signs a form. Then a doctor, usually the person's general practitioner but sometimes a casualty officer if the person is seen in the accident department, signs the medical recommendation. This must be done within twenty-four hours of examining the patient. At this point a second opinion must be offered to the patient and whilst some patients opt for this, others do not. Finally, the psychiatrist is the one who makes the ultimate decision and completes the third section of the form thereby accepting the patient as involuntary. Sometimes the psychiatrist declines to complete the form if the opinion is that admission in these circumstances is not required or if the patient agrees to come to hospital voluntarily. If the patient feels that the detention is illegal then an application can be made for judicial review through the hospital administration or through a solicitor.

Most compulsory admissions are brief and last less than fourteen days because with improvement in the psychiatric condition the person is no longer a threat to self or to others.

No Need for Fear

From this you will see that you have little to fear from your husband and that it would be extremely difficult for him to have you admitted to hospital against your will in the absence of severe psychiatric illness. Psychiatrists are very conscious of patients' rights and a doctor detaining a patient on flimsy grounds could face disciplinary proceedings from the doctors' professional body, the Medical Council, as well as a civil suit for unlawful detention in the courts.

* * *

You are obviously fearful of what your husband is threatening but I suggest that you discuss your fears with your general practitioner and also with your solicitor as a precaution. Ultimately, if your husband continues with these threats you must seriously consider your future with him.

Useful Contact
Irish Council for Civil Liberties
Tel. (01) 6779813

Medico-Legal

My mother, aged seventy-nine, has Alzheimer's dementia, and she made her will two years ago. I wonder if it is valid, as she gave her money to a very unusual charity and her property to a distant cousin in Australia with whom we have had little contact. In her first will she left her estate to me, as she has always lived with me, but subsequently changed her mind when she thought I was trying to poison her. What should I do?

It is very difficult to advise you about a will – you really need legal advice. I suggest you consult your solicitor about this immediately. The ability to make a will is known as testamentary capacity and if a current will is found to be invalid then the previous one becomes valid again. Your solicitor will have to decide if at the time of making her most recent will, the one which you are questioning, she was fully capable of doing so. If her Alzheimer's disease has set in since that will was made, then it is probably still valid. However, if she had well-developed dementia at the time there is a possibility that the most recent will is invalid.

Valid Will

There are three aspects that need to be considered in deciding if a will is valid. Firstly, does the person appreciate the size of their estate? If the person has no knowledge of the size and contents of their estate, due to illness, then the will may be invalid. Of course some very wealthy people are indifferent to the size of their estate but this is a separate matter and is a problem unlikely to assail many.

Secondly, does the person understand the implications of making or changing a will? This means that the person must have a full realisation that in making a will their estate is to be given to the named person or organisation after their death. They must also understand that a will can be changed at any time and that all previous wills are then invalid. The person must also make the will freely and without undue pressure to make particular bequests.

Thirdly, does the person appreciate which people may expect to benefit from his estate? This is one of the areas where your solicitor will need to examine matters very carefully, as in your letter you say that your mother thought you were trying to poison her. Assuming that this was not true, a belief such as this suggests that her understanding of who would benefit from her estate may have been influenced by her illness. Being convinced that you were trying to poison her could have led her to alter her will on the basis of these false beliefs, known as delusions.

Full Assessment

Your solicitor will probably arrange for your mother to be seen medically. He will write for reports from her general practitioner and from other doctors who may have treated her. If your mother's dementia was diagnosed by her general practitioner on clinical grounds alone, he may request that she see a consultant geriatrician or psychiatrist in order to confirm the diagnosis, as severe depression, especially in an elderly person, can also resemble dementia. In addition, brain scans and memory assessments may be required to confirm the diagnosis and the likely date of onset. Surprisingly, the degree of understanding about matters such as property or money does not seem to be related to the extent of the damage to the brain as shown by a scan.

The medical personnel assessing your mother will also be interested to learn about her feelings towards you, particularly her beliefs concerning your behaviour towards her. If at the time of making the will your mother was in the early stages of Alzheimer's disease her will might be valid, as people at this point in the course of the disease often have patches of clear understanding and other times when they are less lucid. The medical evaluation as well as the information obtained from the solicitor who drew up the last will, will be crucial. In particular, they will be asked to outline how she presented to them and whether she appeared to be deluded or confused.

* * *

I hope you clarify the position speedily.

Useful Website

www.efc.ie/publications/legal_updates/articles/priv_client/instructions_elderly_client.html

I was recently caught shoplifting a pair of tights from a shop. I feel terrible that I have disgraced myself and especially my family. I have always tried to be honest – this is so out of character for me. I was already attending my doctor and had commenced treatment for depression – now I really have something to be depressed about. I never thought I would become a kleptomaniac.

I am sorry that this has happened to you; it is clear that you are an honest woman. You may not be aware that shoplifting is one of the symptoms of depressive illness, which you say you were suffering with at the time. You must tell your solicitor about this, as it may be relevant if you are being prosecuted and you must also inform him if you are being treated for depression by a psychologist or psychiatrist. In all probability, your doctor/therapist will then be asked to provide a report on your condition and the contribution, if any, that this made to your shoplifting.

Forgetfulness

Poor concentration and forgetfulness are thought to be behind shoplifting in these circumstances – the person simply forgets that the goods have not been paid for. Research in this area shows that the items are often of little monetary value and are also not of any particular use to the individual who takes them. The episode that you describe certainly fits this pattern, as does the fact that you are female, as shoplifting is more common among women with depression than among men with this condition. Once your depression is adequately treated you will not be at any risk of repeating this.

Telling the Family

You will have to decide whether to tell your husband and family. If you have a good and supportive relationship with them it would be a help to share your feelings about what has happened. However, your own feelings of shame and guilt may prevent you doing this. I suggest that you wait for a little while and your solicitor may be able to indicate the likelihood of a prosecution being taken against you. It is possible that this matter could be resolved without recourse to legal proceedings once the circumstances of the episode are made known. You may then decide that there is no need to inform your family of what has happened. I would advise you to think carefully about this decision.

Not Kleptomania

You use the term kleptomania but I do not believe that you are a kleptomaniac, as it is usually understood. Kleptomania is defined as a recurrent failure to resist impulses to steal objects not needed for personal use or for their monetary value. Before the act there is mounting tension followed by lessening anxiety afterwards. Guilt and feelings of humiliation set in afterwards but during the act there is little thought about being apprehended. The stealing is repetitive and not planned. Unlike other acts of stealing when the aim is to procure the stolen object, kleptomania has as its object the act of stealing. The basis for this repetitive stealing lies deeply rooted in the individual's past. Since your act of stealing was a once off and occurred in the context of depression, you should not regard yourself as a kleptomaniac but as an ill person for whom this unfortunate episode was a symptom.

* * *

I hope that you can quickly put this stressful episode behind you and that you will not continue to blame yourself.

Useful Website

www.psychnet-uk.com/dsm_iv/kleptomania.htm

Useful Contact

AWARE
72 Lower Leeson Street, Dublin 2, Tel. (01) 6617211

Can psychiatric illness be feigned? I have been reading recently that prisoners and army personnel in times past did this so as to avoid imprisonment or conscription.

You are correct in saying that there are descriptions in literature of prisoners and soldiers trying to mimic "madness" so as to avoid unpleasant consequences for themselves. In 1898 the first description of this was written by a psychiatrist called Ganser. He described four criminals who developed very unusual symptoms that were thought at the time to be deliberately contrived. They were giving ridiculous answers to simple questions such as "How many legs has a horse?" The answer given was "Three", indicating that the person understood the question. Other symptoms that were described were disorientation in time (not knowing the day, date etc.), hearing or seeing things that did not exist (hallucinations) and afterwards having no recollection of the period during which these symptoms were observed. This became known as Ganser syndrome. However, many psychiatrists now believe that it is not deliberately contrived at all but that it may have a physical basis due to brain damage, since many who present with these symptoms have a recent history of head injury. Some other authorities suggest that it may in fact be associated with a diagnosis of schizophrenia.

Similar Conditions

There is a type of schizophrenia known as "hebephrenic" schizophrenia that has as its symptoms giggling and silliness as well as muddled sentences due to abnormalities of the thought process. This condition can sometimes give the impression that the person is just making it up and being deliberately childish. This, however, is far from the case and it is a severe form of schizophrenia that in the past had a poor outcome, although this has improved with modern treatment.

There is also a condition known as "hysteria" or conversion disorder in which physical symptoms such as paralysis, blindness, fits etc. occur but without any physical abnormality being detected. In the past it was assumed that the patient must be deliberately faking these symptoms. However, it is now recognised that they are a physical manifestation of overwhelming stress, where the psychic pain is converted into a physical response.

Anxiety and Depression

It is possible, and probably relatively easy, to malinger the milder conditions such as depression, anxiety, post-traumatic stress disorder and phobias, since their diagnosis is based on obtaining a history of symptoms rather than from physical investigations. As information on all psychiatric disorders and their symptoms is now easily accessed on the Internet, the possibility of malingering must be considered in certain circumstances – for example when there is the likelihood of financial gain in association with accidents or with early retirement on the grounds of psychiatric illness etc. This is not to suggest that most people in these circumstances are not genuine but that we should be aware of the possibility. The ability to detect this depends on a thorough history and on getting independent, objective information on the person's functioning.

Standing Trial

A situation in which serious psychiatric illness may be feigned can arise when there is a criminal trial for murder involved and the person may be pleading insanity. In everyday practice, however, it is very rare and can be identified by a period of in-patient assessment. There are also case reports of people feigning memory loss or brain damage so as to avoid court appearances on criminal charges but these too can be easily detected using psychological tools that assess memory and intelligence.

*   *   *

In fact malingering psychiatric illness is not a new phenomenon associated with our "victim" culture but is even described in the Old Testament in the First Book of Samuel (chapter 21, verse 13) when King David feigned madness to escape King Achish of Gath – "So Achish said to his officials 'Look the man is mad! … Haven't I got enough madmen already? Why bring another one to annoy me with his daft actions right here in my own house?"

Useful Website

www.chclibrary.org/micromed/00055920.html

I have a great interest in learning about mental illness and I try to read all I can about it. I am curious to know what the position is when a person with serious mental illness commits a crime such as murder. Surely such a person cannot be held responsible for their actions? Yet I believe that the public should also be protected. Do you have any information on this?

This is indeed a very complex area. You are correct in your observation that whilst a person with serious mental illness cannot always be held responsible for their actions when they commit a serious crime, the public also needs assurances that such a person is in a safe place so that they are protected. Humanitarian concerns would also dictate that such a person should receive appropriate treatment.

M'Naghten Rules

The starting point for understanding the legal position in Ireland when a person with serious psychiatric illness such as manic-depression or schizophrenia takes a life begins with the M'Naghten (pronounced *macnawton*) rules. In 1843, Daniel M'Naghten held a delusional belief that he was being persecuted by the Tory party and that as a consequence his life was in danger. He followed the secretary to the then Prime Minister Sir Robert Peel, whom he mistook for Peel, up Whitehall and shot him in the back; the secretary died five days later. M'Naghten was tried for murder but acquitted on the grounds of insanity. The basis for his acquittal has become known as the M'Naghten Rules and these are now utilised in the courts in Britain and Ireland.

In Britain, the concept of diminished responsibility is also used in certain circumstances, although this does not yet apply in Ireland.

Essential Elements

The central element of the Rules relates to how the person was thinking at the time of the crime. It does not concern itself with how the person is at the time of the trial or prior to the offence. This defence is used when it is argued that the accused, at the time of the crime, was suffering from a "defect of reason" or from a disease of the mind, so as not to know the nature and quality of the act, or that the accused did not know that his actions were wrong. For example, a person may accept that killing another is wrong but under a delusion of persecution may believe he was justified in order to defend himself (as in the original M'Naghten case).

It is important to realise when the cause of delusions or of abnormal behaviours come from outside the person such as the effect of illegal drugs or of alcohol intoxications the M'Naghten Rules do not apply. There is a principle that in these circumstances, since they were self-induced, the person must accept responsibility for their actions. These rules therefore apply when the person has schizophrenia or a similar illness.

Special Verdict

The verdict delivered in those cases where the M'Naghten Rules have been successfully argued is known as the Special Verdict and is summarised as "guilty but insane", although it is proposed under new legislation currently before the Houses of the Oireachtas to change this to "not guilty by reason of insanity". In addition, a new verdict of "guilty but with diminished responsibility" is to be introduced to cover those situations where the behaviour may be due to an external factor such as drugs.

Safety of Others

As you correctly observe it is important to protect the public whilst offering appropriate treatment to those who commit crimes under the influence of mental illness. Following such a verdict the guilty person is transferred to the Central Mental Hospital in Dublin and remains there until the State determines the person no longer poses a threat. The court has no power to determine this and ordinarily the detention lasts for many years. In Britain, the person will be treated in one of the Special Psychiatric Hospitals such as Broadmoor or Rampton.

Fitness to Plead

A matter that is sometimes raised is the person's capacity to stand trial. This requires consideration of the mental state of the accused at the time of the trial rather than at the time of the crime. The elements that are considered are whether they have the capacity to instruct a legal team, to understand the charges, to follow the evidence and to challenge a juror to whom they may object. If it is concluded that the accused cannot plead then the person is returned to the Central Mental Hospital and treated until their fitness to stand trial returns.

* * *

The interface between law, crime and mental illness is an evolving one and came to the fore recently following the murders in Soham, Cambridgeshire, when the accused was taken to a Special Hospital and his capacity to stand trial evaluated over several weeks. It was concluded that he was fit to give evidence. Other high-profile cases in which psychiatric aspects have been to the fore include the Yorkshire Ripper and the Moors Murderers.

Useful Reading

Winchester, Simon (1998) *The Surgeon of Crowthorne*, Penguin Books: London

Useful Websites

www.peterjepson.com/law/insanity.pdf

www.garysturt.free-online.co.uk/crime/couroom.htm

Miscellaneous

Our industrial society is out to satisfy each and every need and our consumer society even creates some needs to satisfy. The most important need, however, the basic need for meaning, remains – more often than not – ignored and neglected.

Viktor Frankl,
The Will to Meaning, *1969*

I am a secondary school teacher and one of my pupils' parents tells me that their child has attention deficit hyperactivity disorder. I know about this condition from in-house training but I don't really understand it. I have also read about it in the media and it seems that many children in America are being diagnosed with this condition. Is it just a fad?

Attention deficit hyperactivity disorder (ADHD) does indeed exist and it is about three times more common in boys than girls. Abnormalities in a brain chemical called dopamine is probably one of the important causes and research using modern scanning techniques show that the brain centres concerned with attention are smaller in children with this condition.

Figures for its prevalence from England confirm that about 1 per cent of school children are so diagnosed; there are no accurate figures from Ireland. However, you are correct in your concern that it may be a fashionable fad. In the United States, figures suggest that 2–20 per cent of school children have this condition. This wide variation raises concern. It may mean that children who are simply misbehaving and undisciplined are being given this label.

Delayed Diagnosis

Due to its symptoms this disorder is often not diagnosed and parents may think that their child is bold. Others may believe that the child's disorganisation is due to a lack of structure to the day. One of the characteristic features is that the child does not respond to the usual disciplinary rules of the household or school, so social graces such as not interrupting, no matter how often stated, are ignored. This may lead parents to assume that they are not disciplining their child properly and so the child's condition remains undiagnosed well into their schooling.

Two Types

There are two types of ADHD, although with some overlap: the inattention type and the more common hyperactive type. Those with inattention-type ADHD have difficulty concentrating and focussing. They tend to be very forgetful and so will lose school books, clothes etc. to an extraordinary degree. This will be very noticeable in the classroom: their homework will be either not done or incomplete and they will dive into exams with great enthusiasm but only answer some of the questions. The more noticeable hyperactive-type ADHD is very disruptive, as these children are "on the go" non-stop. They cannot sit still, they fidget constantly and they sleep very little. They also have great difficulty concentrating and tend to be explosively irritable even to minor triggers. This may dismay their classmates. However, they are also very sensitive and easily moved to laughter or tears.

All of these features lead to major educational and social difficulties for the child if untreated. Classmates shun them, they become friendless and their self-worth plummets. Their impulsivity and irritability can lead them into conflict with the law and some may end up in prison.

Treatable

Fortunately, this is a treatable condition once it is diagnosed. The most commonly used medication is Ritalin, which is effective in up to three-quarters of children, but others are also available. Ritalin is only licensed for use in those under the age of 16 in Ireland but is available for all ages in Britain. A recent study found that about 75 per cent of children on Ritalin showed a significant improvement on their classroom performance; self-confidence also improves when the child is no longer being constantly reprimanded. The importance of the school in monitoring progress with treatment is obvious. Sometimes medication is discontinued during school holidays.

By late adolescence the condition improves significantly in many and by the mid-twenties it will have burnt itself out in most, even without treatment, due to the increase in volume that occurs in brain cells as they mature. Unfortunately, for some, this will be too late due to the behavioural, social and academic consequences.

* * *

Treatment will not make any difference to pre-existing learning difficulties nor will it turn the child into a perfect child. It is important in the classroom to have the same expectations of the child as of any other pupil and so excuses such as "It's my ADD" are not acceptable. The successfully treated child will display the same behaviours as any other child and will need to be disciplined or rewarded in the same way.

Useful Reading

Oireachtas Subcommittee report on Attention Deficit Disorder, available from the Department of Health

Useful Website

www.chadd.org

I am thirty years old and have recently got married. My wife seems to be very suspicious of me, especially when I talk to other women. I try to reassure her that she is the only one I love by buying her presents. I have also asked friends to reassure her that I am not being unfaithful. In spite of this she seems to misinterpret everything I do, even when I talk casually to female colleagues. Initially I was flattered by her attention but now I am beginning to feel that it is very claustrophobic. Are my feelings normal?

It is quite normal to feel that the constant preoccupation of your wife is suffocating. It is often common for very young women, or men, to be jealous, particularly those who are insecure. Like you, many initially feel flattered by being the focus of attention and by the knowledge that they are so desired by another as to be possessed by them. However, once the teenage years have passed, most people will realise that such attention is unhealthy. It is perfectly normal to talk with others, be they colleagues from work, previous girlfriends or neighbours.

Trust

Relationships are built on mutual trust and on the belief that past relationships or friendships do not interfere with love for one's spouse. If your relationship with your wife is based on having to prove your fidelity rather than on trust, serious questions need to be asked and answered. It is likely that your wife will rationalise her behaviour by saying that when couples love each other they have no secrets or that they should become mutually dependent. This enmeshment is very unhealthy.

Collusion

I would suggest that you stop involving your friends in her doubts and that you tell her that from now on she must accept the truth of your love unconditionally, without the necessity for constant reassurance, as do most other couples. It may seem that this is very hard, since it is the most natural thing in the world to try to reassure another about your love. However, by providing constant reassurance you are reinforcing her doubt in you and it is likely that the effect of the reassurance will be short lived. Why not say something like "I know you doubt me but from now on you must take my love on trust, as I take yours on trust".

Reason for this Jealousy?

Jealousy such as this has been written about by Shakespeare in his tragedy *Othello*. It deals with the overwhelming jealousy of Othello for his wife and of her death as a result. This pattern of jealousy has come to be known as the Othello syndrome.

Sometimes jealousy is associated with excessive alcohol consumption, which can either cause the jealousy or worsen it if the tendency already exists. If your wife is drinking to excess this should be strongly discouraged. Also, if there is any misuse of illegal drugs such as cannabis, amphetamines or cocaine the jealousy may increase. Occasionally, it may be part of a more serious psychiatric illness, such as schizophrenia.

If you have experienced any violence or any bizarre behaviour, such as searching your pockets for "evidence" of infidelity, then the problem is even more serious than you have outlined and may require professional help from a psychiatrist. A legal remedy may ultimately be necessary.

The outcome of therapy is generally not good if the jealousy is intrinsic to the person. However, if the jealousy is clearly linked to alcohol or drug misuse, the prognosis can be better. The effectiveness of therapy is also linked to the insight that the person has, since the belief that the mistrust is justified may be difficult to alter.

* * *

I recommend that you and your wife seek urgent help before it gets out of control and your marriage becomes a battleground. Hopefully the jealousy will pass as your wife matures but if it does not then you must be prepared to consider all options for your marriage, including separation.

Useful Contacts

ACCORD
Tel. (01) 4780866

MRCS (Marriage and Relationship Counselling Services)
Tel. (01) 6799341

My son's marriage broke up last year. He was feeling a bit depressed afterward but he's fine again. However, he has become very religious recently. He has started going to church again, for the first time in years, and he is planning a retreat in a monastery. I'm pleased in one sense but I'm also concerned as it is so unlike him and I wonder if he could have "religious mania". I would hate to see him becoming fanatical.

I am sure you are surprised at this change in your son and understandably you are trying to comprehend what is happening. When people have traumas in their lives, such as your son had when his marriage broke up, they often re-evaluate their lives and decide that spiritual rather than material things are important. This may have been the catalyst for your son's re-involvement with religion. Also, people often tell me that when they are depressed they turn to prayer as a comfort but also as a way of trying to do something about their predicament. Praying may not seem like "doing" but when the hopelessness of depression is dominating life then praying and asking for help does indeed seem like doing something. In those circumstances people also feel that they are being "listened to" and they get comfort from believing there is a power greater than themselves. So your son's re-involvement with religious practice is not all that unusual in the circumstances.

Religious Mania

I am unsure what you mean by the term "religious mania", as it is not a medical term. Perhaps you are concerned that your son may have some serious psychiatric illness that is causing him to be more religious than is normal for him. It is true that some psychiatric illnesses such as schizophrenia or manic-depression, especially in the high or manic phase, are associated with excessive religious fervour. Also, when people are very depressed they often believe they are guilty of serious sins or that they deserve punishment. If there are any indications of over-activity, excessive spending of money, hearing voices or getting unusual beliefs, for example that he is the Messiah or a saint, then the possibility of psychiatric illnesses should be considered. However, your son would certainly be talking about these things to you as they are almost impossible to conceal. So it is very unlikely, although not impossible, that major psychiatric illness is the explanation.

You have mentioned that you would hate to see your son becoming fanatical. A fanatic is a person whose enthusiasm is extreme or beyond the norm. It does not sound like this is the case with your son. For example, if he had never stopped practising his religion, would you have this worry now? Is what he is doing so unusual that in ordinary circumstances you would be troubled by it?

If the answer is no, then it would appear that your concern stems from this being a change in pattern for him rather than because it is alarming in itself.

I suggest you speak with your son and perhaps begin by telling him how pleased you are that he appears to be feeling better. You can then mention your surprise at his new-found interest in religion and he might well tell you what is behind it. However, you should not interrogate him, as spiritual matters are often very private; if your son has gone through some type of religious experience, he may be reluctant to share it with anybody at present.

A priest might also be able to advise you, since they are very familiar with the difference between fanaticism and healthy religious belief and practice.

* * *

There is a substantial body of psychiatric research showing the benefits of religion in protecting against some types of emotional disorder, especially depression. And of course it can help protect against self-harm. Therefore, I would not be concerned about your son's new-found interest in his old religion and I think you should give him space to develop it as he feels appropriate.

Useful Reading

Jamison, Kay Redfield (1979) *An Unquiet Mind*, Vintage Books: New York

Useful Website

www.psychiatrictimes.com/p001078.html

I am hoping to work with refugees and asylum seekers for a few weeks as part of my college course. I am sure life must be very difficult for them in a strange country and I wonder if they have any particular emotional or psychological problems of which I should be aware? It is so difficult to get this information anywhere.

There is great credit due to you for showing this interest in and sensitivity to immigrants to our country. Unfortunately, there is no research from Ireland on this topic, but there is a significant amount from Britain that can inform us.

Language

One of the major difficulties is diagnosing emotional problems in this group of people. Obviously, many may not speak English fluently and so actually describing clearly what they are feeling can be difficult. This is surmountable provided interpreters can be found, but it may delay diagnosis and it can mean that serious psychiatric illness then presents as an emergency.

For cultural reasons that are specific to them, and because they have not had the same media exposure to psychological jargon as we have, asylum seekers and refugees may describe their distress very differently than we do. Many do not have a language for emotional distress and instead express it in physical terms. This is known as "alexythymia", which means that instead of presenting with feelings of tension, sadness or anxiety, they may describe symptoms such as "a heavy heart", soreness in the chest or headache. The fact that they may attend their doctor with physical symptoms may delay accurate diagnosis and they may be referred for physical tests initially.

Grieving

An added burden for many to bear will be the sadness they feel at leaving their loved ones in the home country. This is most likely to be a serious problem for those who have come seeking asylum, since they may have had to leave in a hurry, unable to say their goodbyes. Some of them may also have lost family members during war and if the bodies have not been recovered then this will be an added source of distress for them. Therefore, many asylum seekers and refugees will have complicated grief reactions for which they will require professional help. However, grief may be expressed in a very different way from what we are used to, making it difficult to identify abnormal grief reactions. In addition, their funeral rituals may be very different from ours and so our bereavement counsellors may not yet have the culturally appropriate skills to help them.

Post-Traumatic Stress Disorder

Many asylum seekers and refugees will have experienced violence and torture and may have seen others being killed or maimed. Post-traumatic stress disorder is therefore likely to be a huge problem and having suitably trained therapists who speak their language is vital, although we may not always have such a resource available.

Local Problems

Unfortunately, many asylum-seekers and refugees are unemployed. In any culture unemployment is associated with a variety of psychiatric disorders, particularly stress-related and depressive disorders. Similarly, if they are resented by the local population and are socially isolated then they will also be at heightened risk of emotional problems, as is anybody in such a situation.

Khat

Although many migrants do not drink alcohol because of religious sanctions, there may be problems with illicit drugs that heretofore we have not seen in Ireland. Khat (pronounced "cot") is derived from a plant of that name and is grown in the Horn of Africa. In London this is sold by greengrocers and is chewed or made into tea. It is popular among emigrants from Somalia, the Yemen and Ethiopia. It remains to be seen if it becomes a problem here but it is important to be aware of the possibility. Similar to amphetamines it increases alertness, reduces appetite and can cause irritability and violence in some along with craving and deep depression when it is stopped. It is also associated with thirst and produces a strong aroma.

* * *

Asylum seekers and refugees present specific and challenging mental health problems and it is unclear if our services in Ireland are equipped to respond to these. The work of volunteers such as you will be one further asset to this group of deprived people.

Useful Reading

"Refugees and Primary Care: Tackling the Inequalities", *BMJ*, 1998, 317:1444–1446 (November 21st)
(This is available online by visiting a search engine and keying in BMJ)

Useful Contact

Refugee Council of Ireland
40 Lower Dominic Street, Dublin 1, Tel. (01) 8730042

My wife suffers with very bad rheumatoid arthritis and has been put on steroids by her consultant. To my horror I discovered that these drugs can cause depression and as she was already feeling very low when she started them, I am worried that she will get even more depressed. Are there any other psychological problems caused by these drugs? I have told her to stop taking them and get something else from her doctor.

On no account should your wife stop taking these drugs unless it is done under medical supervision, as this could cause major problems that are sometimes fatal. If she has stopped them she should contact her doctor immediately, as this would definitely be regarded as a medical emergency.

Feeling Depressed

One of the problems that your wife faces is that she is already low in mood. This does not necessarily mean that she has a clinical depression requiring treatment in its own right. It may be that her mood is low for the very understandable reason that she has a painful and incapacitating illness that makes her less agile than before. In particular, if she has never had a problem with depression in the past, there is a strong possibility that your wife's low mood is a response to her altered physical state. If the steroids help her arthritis then I would expect her mood to improve.

Moodiness

As you point out, steroids can cause psychological changes, making the person moody and changeable. For example, she may be in very good form one day, but be tearful and irritable the next. This moodiness is generally unrelated to changes in physical well-being. Some people describe insomnia with these drugs, again not due to discomfort or pain but for no obvious reason. Other more prolonged mood changes can occur, accompanied by poor concentration, tearfulness and loss of interest in the usual activities and hobbies. This is a full-blown clinical depression secondary to the medication rather than an understandable reaction to the pain of the illness. These mood changes are the most common psychological side effects.

Generally, these effects occur in the first few days of treatment and if the medication is reduced or stopped the symptoms improve. It may not be possible to do this if the benefits to the physical illness outweigh those of psychological well-being. In these circumstances, the depressive episode will require treatment in its own right with antidepressants.

Less Common Effects

Other less common effects on mood occur, in particular a false rise in mood that may seem inappropriate to the circumstances. This elation or hypomania is also associated with loss of sleep, racing thoughts, speech that is rapid and pressured and a requirement for less sleep than usual. As with depression, elation, if it is going to occur, happens in the first week or so of treatment. This can be controlled by tailoring the dose of steroid that is prescribed or by adding a specific treatment to control the elation.

Other uncommon side effects are paranoia or suspiciousness. Very rarely confusion is present and the person is unable to describe what is currently in the news, or give the day, date and so on. This passes when the steroids are reduced or discontinued. You should read the patient information leaflet that now comes with all medications.

Past History

These side effects are more likely to occur when the person receiving steroids has a past history of these conditions. If your wife has no such history then the risk of her getting these effects is less than those who have a history of depression, elation or manic-depression. If she has such a history her doctor should be told in order that treatment can be tailored accordingly.

*　*　*

I hope that your wife responds well to the treatment and if she does I expect her old self will emerge again.

Useful Website

www.drrichardhall.com/steroid.htm

I have recently learnt that my nephew in England has a psychiatric condition, that he has been an in-patient and is now taking medication prescribed by a psychiatrist. He is well again and back at work and wants to come to me for a holiday, as we have always been close. He says he wants to talk to me about his illness. However, I'm terrified that he may become violent or behave unpredictably. What should I do?

Most violent incidents are committed by those in the general population who are deemed to be "normal". Even the most serious crimes such as rape and murder are usually perpetrated, not by psychiatric patients, but by family members and others known to the victim. Numerous studies have demonstrated this, although the few murders that have been committed by psychiatric patients have been very high profile.

Stigma

Your reaction is similar to that of many people who are confronted with psychiatric disorder. Unfortunately, those with emotional problems are stigmatised and the public has some unusual ideas about how they may react. You have no need to fear that your nephew will become violent – this is one of the myths that abounds.

Sometimes if a serious psychiatric disorder is untreated or if the prescribed medicines are not taken and the person relapses, aggressive behaviour may become evident – this is occasional and not commonplace. However, once appropriate treatment is reinstated the aggression settles. In such circumstances it is best to avoid confrontation rather than try to negotiate, as these volatile situations, like any hostile situation, can escalate.

In fact, the aggression that those with psychiatric disorders exhibit is more usually directed to themselves in the form of self-harm or, even more tragically, completed suicide. For example, about 10 per cent of those who are alcoholic die by suicide and about 7 per cent of those with depressive illness, manic-depression or schizophrenia end their lives.

Good News

It is wonderful that your nephew is so well again and he is to be strongly encouraged to continue taking his treatment. Provided he remains well the chances of a violent outburst are no higher than if he never had any problems at all. Far from being fearful of him you should be celebrating his well-being

Miscellaneous 149

and most definitely inviting him to stay. To reassure yourself, you could talk with his parents if they are willing.

When he does visit you he should avoid alcohol, since it can lead to a depressed mood very rapidly and can also interact badly with some medications. This might result in him becoming drowsy and having difficulty driving. Adequate sleep is also very important for those recovering from psychiatric disorder. It goes without saying also that cannabis or other recreational drugs should definitely be avoided for the same reason.

Respect

Your nephew should be treated no differently than any other member of your family with the above caveats in mind. If he does speak with you about the details of his illness you should respect his confidentiality. It is important that you do not start exploring with him what did or did not cause his illness, since this requires the expertise of a mental health professional. It is also vital he be reassured that psychiatric disorders are not a sign of weakness but that they are illnesses just like diabetes or high blood pressure. Lifestyle may occasionally play a part but it would be a dangerous over-simplification to assume that this is the case with your nephew.

* * *

You should provide a listening ear and support his decision to continue to attend a psychiatrist. Have no fear; it is wonderful that he is well enough to want to share his healing with you.

Useful Contacts

GROW
(Community Mental Health Movement)
167 Capel Street, Dublin 1, Tel. (01) 8734029

RECOVERY
Cherry Orchard Hospital, Dublin 10, Tel. (01) 6260775

Changing Minds
(Anti-stigma campaign)
Irish Division, Royal College of Psychiatrists, 17 Belgrave Square, London, SW1X 8PG, Tel. (01) 4022346

Why do psychiatrists give medication for everything? What about counselling? Surely if we dealt with the causes of problems then people wouldn't be in and out of hospital all the time.

Unfortunately, many people hold this view and believe that psychiatrists use nothing but medication. There is a mistaken view that medication is not necessary and that we prescribe it only because we have not got the time to talk or listen to our patients. This is a fundamental misunderstanding. We adhere to what is termed a "bio-psycho-social" view of psychiatric illness, which means that in psychiatric illnesses there are biological, psychological and social elements, all of which need to be addressed. For each patient the mix of these elements varies.

Different Elements

This means that the relative strength of each of these three components will determine the approach to treatment. For some patients it may be exclusively a talking therapy, for others a behavioural therapy and for others still medication may be the principal treatment. Many patients require several approaches. For example, with a person who has a phobia of dogs triggered by being bitten as a child there will be a large psychological element (the fear resulting from the bite), a negligible biological element and, if they have been encouraged to avoid dogs as a result, a large social element maintaining the fear. Treatment will therefore focus on the psychological element with behaviour therapy and on the social element. However, with a person suffering from schizophrenia there is a large biological element and any medications that are used must have been shown in trials to be effective for the biological component of the disorder. If relationships at home are poor there may also be a social component worsening the illness, and treatment will then use both medication and family therapy.

Repeat Admissions

You seem to be suggesting that medication cannot be very helpful since patients have repeated admissions. However, it is important to realise that only a small fraction of those attending a psychiatrist need to come into hospital – of the order of 15 per cent. Many of those who require medication do not accept that they need it and do not take it as prescribed; others begin to take their treatment but stop taking it when they feel well. Overall only about 30 per cent of patients take medication as prescribed; this is little different from the pattern among patients attending physicians and general practitioners. Around

70 per cent of admissions to psychiatric units are due to relapse as a result of failure to take medication as prescribed. This is also a problem with talking treatments, with patients often failing to attend their appointments, dropping out when it becomes challenging or not carrying out the between-therapy exercises.

Treating the Causes

On the face of it trying to deal with the triggers to illnesses has intuitive appeal. It is, unfortunately, a complicated area. Suppose a person smokes very heavily and gets bronchitis. While tackling the cause, i.e. smoking, is vital, it is also important to treat each acute attack of bronchitis with antibiotics to prevent worsening of the condition. Psychiatric illnesses are similar in that triggers and risk factors if present must be addressed. However, once an illness has occurred it must be treated in its own right. Thereafter, there is a biological vulnerability to recurrences for some of the conditions such as schizophrenia and depression. Some talking treatments when combined with medication can reduce this risk and may eventually allow for its discontinuation, but others continue to be at risk and require long-term medication even after they have had talking therapy.

Of course helping the person deal with underlying problems is very important, at a human level. In some instances this may prevent recurrences but there is no guarantee. This is because some of these background problems are risk factors for illness – in other words they do not trigger the illness but increase the chance of becoming ill and may not be remediable, for example the loss of a mother in childhood. Finally, it is important to recognise that not everybody has a trigger for an illness and that sometimes illness can develop out of the blue.

***

So the role of medication and talking treatments is complex and depends on the mix of biological, psychological and social factors as well as on the person's type of vulnerability and triggers.

Useful Website

www.critpsynet.freeuk.com/Gilbert.htm

Personality Disorders

Surely everybody has a personality disorder to some extent. Nobody is perfect.

Common myth

Personality Disorders

I live with my parents but I have been having huge problems with them recently. We argue all the time and I get very down. As a result I have begun to drink heavily and I took an overdose a few weeks ago. I was referred to a psychiatrist and was told I had a borderline personality disorder and that there was no treatment. I never before heard of this condition. A friend said it might be like manic-depression.

I am sorry that you have been having problems at home and that you have been depressed and drinking. Borderline personality disorder is a controversial diagnosis and there is disagreement about what it really is.

Multiple Symptoms

Some psychiatrists believe borderline personality disorder to be a condition that lies on the border of the psychoses – those conditions in which there is loss of contact with reality. According to that view, your friend is partly correct, since manic-depression is one of the psychotic disorders and the other is schizophrenia. However, this view of borderline personality disorder is an old one and no longer holds sway.

In its modern meaning it is a description of personality traits and behaviours that are persistent from adolescence and through adulthood and include depressed mood, poor self-esteem, impulsive behaviour, often associated with repeated self-harm such as overdosing and fear of being abandoned. Some people also describe feelings of emptiness and have very intense relationships, alternating between hostility and love. Sometimes there is also difficulty in controlling anger and there may be periods of memory loss and eating problems.

No single one of these features is enough to make the diagnosis and they have to be present throughout life rather than on the very odd occasion or when under particular stress, as you seem to be under at present.

Improvement

Some experts in the past believed that this condition could develop into schizophrenia, but recent studies show that this does not happen. In fact, the good news is that it improves as the sufferer matures and learns better styles of coping. The diagnosis is rarely made in anybody over the age of forty, since by then stability and better relationships will have been achieved.

However, if alcohol abuse is part of the early pattern of behaviour this may persist and the episodes of depression can also persist into late adulthood. In spite of the difficulty making the diagnosis and the scepticism concerning its existence American studies suggest that it is present in 2 per cent of the population. Those studies also show that many of the sufferers have been sexually abused in childhood.

Treatment

Your psychiatrist is partly correct when she says there is no treatment. Psychotherapy can be effective but it takes several years to bring about improvement. Sometimes focusing on background problems, especially abuse, if present, is more appropriate but again it will take a long time to achieve the goal of coming to terms with what has happened. The depression that accompanies borderline personality disorder often does not respond well to antidepressants. Recently there has been more focus on treating the episodes of self-harm that are part of this condition and a type of behaviour therapy, called dialectic behaviour therapy, has been found helpful in preventing further episodes. Most people just seem to "grow out of it" with maturation.

Premature Diagnosis

I am surprised that this diagnosis has been made in your case, as it is a difficult to do this after a single assessment. Normally, such a label would not be given unless there was evidence over several assessments of the symptoms and behaviours that make up the condition. Of itself, an episode of self-harm is not enough to make the diagnosis and from your letter this seems to be a symptom of your distress about your family rather than part of an established pattern.

You certainly need help, as dealing with problems by over-dosing in clearly not healthy. You might consider asking your parents to meet your psychiatrist or attending for family therapy with them. This might be a better forum for exploring your difficulties rather than having rows that culminate in dangerous behaviours.

I am sorry that you have been labelled after a single meeting. Perhaps you should raise this with your doctor also. If you are not being offered treatment or you remain unhappy with your diagnosis you should approach your general practitioner or your psychiatrist for a second opinion – this is something that most doctors are eager for, especially when a patient is dissatisfied.

* * *

I hope your difficulties can be resolved and that your relationship with your family is restored.

Useful Reading

Paul T. Mason and Kreger, Randi (1998) *Stop Walking on Eggshells: Taking your Life Back when someone you Care about has Borderline Personality Disorder*, New Harbinger Publications: Oakland, CA

Useful Website

www.psycom.net/depression.central.borderline.html

What is multiple personality disorder? I work with a woman whom we all find very difficult. She changes on a daily basis. One day she can be very friendly; the next she is hostile and silent. Even her clothes and style of dressing are unpredictable. I have tried, unsuccessfully, to befriend her. She is a real Jekyll and Hyde character. My colleagues and I wonder if she has multiple personality disorder. I recently read a very interesting article about it. What is this condition?

Multiple personality disorder, also called dissociative identity disorder, is a condition that has huge public appeal and has been the subject of several bestsellers and box-office successes. Interestingly, there are no more than three hundred case reports in the psychiatric literature and most of those have appeared in the past twenty years. This is a surprisingly low number considering that the condition was first described in the United States in 1816, and it is from there and Canada that almost all of these reports have come.

Main Features

Whilst sudden and dramatic changes in personality are the central feature, the other symptoms of the disorder differ from those that you describe in your colleague. In the classic descriptions, each personality has a fully integrated and detailed set of memories, attitudes and behaviours. Each "alternate", as the individual personalities are called, is unaware of the behaviours and traits of the other (hence the term dissociative). In some reports, up to sixty different personalities are reported to reside in one person, although the average is thirteen.

Personalities may be of different gender and often contrast with each other: for example one may be shy, another gregarious and so on. Sometimes they have names that reflect their basic traits, for example "the helper". The "host" personality, the one that carries the legal name, presents for treatment usually of depression or anxiety. It is during treatment that the various alternates emerge, often under the influence of drug-assisted interviews, but sometimes spontaneously. It is believed that this condition is intimately linked to sexual abuse in childhood.

Mechanism

Many psychiatrists and psychologists are sceptical of this diagnostic label, especially in Europe, and maintain that the diagnosis comes about as result of a dominant therapist who suggests that the changeability in mood described by the patient is a manifestation of "multiples". This then further encourages the development of the discreet behaviour found in each personality. Interestingly, there have been no cases documented in the medical literature where the patient did not possess prior knowledge of the condition. However, those who support the diagnosis of multiple personality disorder say that it is becoming increasingly common, due to increased awareness of the disorder itself and the increased recognition of sexual abuse. The latter was the backdrop in popular books dealing with this subject, such as *The Three Faces of Eve* (1957).

Many investigators have tried to identify tangible features that distinguish the different personalities but none so far has been successful. For example, brain tracing – known as EEG – as well as personality tests have failed to differentiate the personalities from each other.

Legal Implications

The diagnosis carries huge legal implications and it was used in the attempted defence of the "Hillside Strangler" – a multiple murderer in Los Angeles in 1979. It was dropped after it was found out that the defendant had previously impersonated a psychologist and had access to his case-notes during psychological evaluation. Other attempts to raise it as a defence have also been unsuccessful.

The argument is that if each personality is separate and has amnesia for the actions of others, how can the host or main personality be held responsible? However, if each personality is separate then the host personality lacks the capacity to decide right from wrong in all circumstances and surely preventive detention might be indicated. At a more mundane level it also raises questions about the capacity to contract a marriage, to open a bank account and so on, since each personality is separate and unknown to the others.

* * *

Since your colleague at work seems to be moody and difficult, but nothing more, it is extremely unlikely that she has multiple personality disorder. If she did, it would be very serious indeed.

Useful Reading
Thiggen, C.H. and Cleckley, H. (1957) *The Three Faces of Eve*, Secker and Warburg: London

Useful Website
www.skepdic.com/mpd.html

I am twenty-five and my partner of eighteen months is very violent. He hits me and drinks a lot. He says he is sorry but then seems to forget just as quickly. He recently attended a psychiatrist who told him that he was a psychopath. I am very worried as we have a baby. What exactly is this condition and can it be cured? I always thought this was a "made-up" term and that such people did not really exist. Will our child be like his father when he grows up?

Unfortunately, psychopaths do exist and are found in all walks of life. This is also part of a recognised psychiatric group of conditions, known as personality disorders. A psychopath is a person who behaves in a callous way without regard for the feelings or needs of others. There is generally an inner coldness and some commit serious crimes, although it is a mistake to assume that every criminal is also a psychopath. Although the psychopathic person appreciates the rules of society, they have little capacity to conform to these and generally choose to ignore them. Many drink to excess and have a very low tolerance for frustration or boredom. Overall, this disorder is much more common among men than women. It is present in all cultures. However, there is a suggestion from research that it is increasing in Western cultures in the last two decades and studies have found that 2–3 per cent of the population have the condition.

No Remorse

One of the key features of this disorder is the inability to learn from experience, so that although punishment may be the consequence of the behaviour, the psychopath still repeats the same actions. Apologies are superficial and there is little genuine remorse or guilt. You must ask yourself if your partner fits this description.

It is also true that many blame others for their behaviour or explain it away by describing themselves a "hard but honest". Regrettably, because of a low boredom threshold, sustaining regular employment or a long-term relationship is very difficult. However, on the surface there is charm and a new acquaintance may feel flattered by the attention and compliments.

Nature versus Nurture

You are rightly concerned that your child might become like his father. There is little research into the genetics of psychopathy, but what is available suggests that a predisposition to this behaviour is inherited. However, there is no certainty that this will in fact happen, as with the right parenting skills this risk can be minimised. In other words, nurture is more powerful than nature.

You should therefore concentrate your efforts on bringing up a child who has consistency in his life in relation to love, discipline and right and wrong.

Changes with Age

Psychopathy is not easily treated, as the origins of the condition lie in childhood experiences, especially exposure to aggressive behaviour during the early years. In addition many will have a long history, even in childhood, of conduct problems, so cruelty to animals, exclusion from school, fighting and vandalism will have been reported. Unlearning this lengthy pattern of behaviour is understandably very difficult. There is no "magic bullet" cure. The limited treatments that are available focus on specific areas such as anger management and problem solving so that impulsiveness is reduced. However, as the person gets older the aggressive behaviour lessens and it may be easier to live with them. This change does not generally take place before the age of forty-five, so there can be years of violence and callousness for family members.

* * *

I am sorry that this may not be what you want to hear, but it is important that you have a full understanding of your predicament at this time, especially for your child's sake.

Useful Website

www.personalitydisorders.mentalhelp.net

(*Psychological Self-Help* by C.E. Tucker-Ladd is available on this website)

I am very interested in psychological/psychiatric issues. I often read in the newspapers, particularly in the section dealing with courts, that a person charged with a crime has been found to have a psychopathic personality disorder. What does this mean? Surely everybody to some extent has a personality disorder, as nobody is perfect?

You are quite right in your observation that nobody is perfect and that we all have abnormal traits. However, personality disorder is quite different from the problematic traits that we all possess. An individual with a personality disorder possesses a cluster of traits, present since early adulthood and often even since childhood, that leads them into repeated interpersonal difficulties with others, particularly those outside the family. The difficulties are not just brief or isolated, such as the occasional argument, but must be serious enough to cause major problems. If you consider this definition you will see that only a small number of people have these features. Studies of personality disorder have found that about 10–15 per cent of the population are so affected. Unlike psychiatric disorders such as depression, which the person can identify as having a clear onset, those with personality disorder are aware of problems from an early age so that it seems the person has never really been free from the associated difficulties.

Types of Personality Disorder

The term "personality disorder" is not a very good one as it sounds almost like a criticism and conjures up images of violence and antisocial behaviour – it is in this regard that you have probably come across the term in the courts. However, besides this antisocial type, or psychopathic type as it was once called, there are other types of personality disorder that are not in any way associated with violence. These never come before the courts except in some cases of civil annulment where the personality problems might be considered as grounds for annulling a marriage.

Some of the types of personality disorder that have been identified include the dependent type, the obsessional type and the anxious type. Those with dependent personality disorder have difficulty making day-to-day decisions without the assistance of others and require constant reassurance, as their self-confidence is very low. This may place great strain on a relationship as a result. In a work situation they may have similar problems and are often taken advantage of and become the butt of bullying. Far from being violent, they are very sad and lonely.

Those who have an obsessional personality are very rigid and fixed in their ways so that even making an unexpected visit on them causes great anxiety

Personality Disorders

and difficulty coping. These are the people who cannot face change, even when it is positive, such as promotion at work.

Those in the anxious group worry constantly about simple things and avoid social situations. They have to be protected from even minor stress, since they decompensate in various psychiatric disorders easily. However, there is overlap between these various groups so it is rare to find a purely anxious or dependent person – rather there will be features of several types mixed together.

Antisocial

It is clear that the antisocial category is one of many and it is found in about 1 per cent of the general population. Its features include violent behaviour and failure to learn from mistakes so that the violent behaviours are repeated. There is no guilt and no feeling of concern for others. Family members often report that they observed aggression and cruelty to animals even during childhood. Not surprisingly, as you observe, these people commit violent crime and come before the courts. They often have alcohol-related problems. The good news is that as time goes by most of those with antisocial behaviour will mature out of this behaviour, although they may have caused great suffering along the way.

In general, personality disorder is difficult to treat but in recent years assertiveness courses, anger management and problem-solving techniques have been used with some success. Unlike most other behavioural and emotional problems, very little has been written to help those with these problems or their families, except in the professional literature, and there are no support organisations that I know of.

* * *

The abnormal traits that we all possess, as you observe, do not lead to the serious problems outlined above and the difficulties that we all experience with others from time to time resolve quickly. It is important not to confuse these normal day-to-day problems with personality disorder.

Useful Reading

Lindenfield, Gael (1992) *Assert Yourself*, Thorsons: London

Psychiatric Services

Carers are an integral part of the patient's support system ... They are the ones with the day-to-day experience of the patient's condition, and they carry the most intimate responsibility for the patient's welfare ... The carer's voice in decision making about admission and discharge is ignored at everyone's peril – and yet so often is.

Dr Mike Shooter,
President, Royal College of Psychiatrists,
Speaking at launch of "Partners in Care" campaign,
January, 2004

My family doctor has suggested that I see a psychiatrist as I have been feeling anxious for the past three months, for no reason, and I don't seem to be getting any better. I am absolutely terrified, as I have often heard it said that psychiatrists are peculiar. Also, I worry that I will be "analysed" and that the things I say will be turned around as if they have a hidden meaning. Perhaps I should see a counsellor instead.

Unfortunately, there are a lot of myths about psychiatrists and one of them is that we are an odd and strange lot! However, this is far from true and most of us are the same as any doctor you might attend. We have families, homes, likes and dislikes and have the same faults and weaknesses as any other group of doctors. It used be said that we had the highest suicide rate in the medical profession, but recent studies suggest this is not the case.

Analysis

Many people assume that we go about analysing them when we meet them socially or professionally, as you suggest. This too is incorrect. Psychoanalysis is a very specific approach to treatment that is not used much at present, since it is very time-consuming and of limited applicability. Analysing people is much more complicated than just looking at them and magically knowing what they think and feel. So your fear that what you say will be scrutinised in some magical way is misplaced.

It is true that we are trained to pick up on body language, so that if, for example, a person becomes tense while speaking about some matter, this will remind us to explore it further. However, this skill is one that is common to clinical psychologists, counsellors, therapists or any mental health professional dealing with the emotions.

First Consultation

When you see the psychiatrist you will not be on a couch, as is sometimes believed, but sitting in a chair as you would in your general practitioner's surgery. The initial consultation will last about forty-five to fifty minutes and an interview with a close family member may also be requested. This is to obtain additional information about the effect your symptoms and problems are having on your day-to-day functioning and relationships. In addition, it will enable an assessment of the kind of person you have always been and hope to return to, from somebody who knows you well.

As you can appreciate, we are often too bound up in our problems to be able to accurately assess the effect they are having on us and on those who are in contact with us. For this reason it is important to speak with somebody who may be more objective. Your psychiatrist is bound by the rules of confidentiality when speaking with this person so you need have no worry that your diagnosis, history or problems will be disclosed without your permission. If you do not want your psychiatrist to speak with a family member you have the absolute right to veto this consultation.

Your History

During the consultation the psychiatrist will ask you about your present problems and the symptoms you are experiencing. You will be asked about your family, your childhood, your education and employment, and your marriage and other relationships. Some regard this as intrusive, but it is important to recognise that past events may make one vulnerable to emotional difficulties in the future and this information can then assist in treatment decisions. For example, if the patient was bereaved in childhood and had not come to terms with the loss, this might require an intervention to help in overcoming the loneliness and sadness that eventually resulted in the current symptoms.

When the consultation is completed you will be told the diagnosis and treatment will be recommended. This will not necessarily be a drug treatment but whatever is suggested you should feel free to ask about duration, side effects and so on. Remember that you are the person with the problem and it is your prerogative to ask questions that you feel are pertinent without feeling guilty. If you have doubts about the treatment being offered it is important to raise these also.

General Practitioner

A letter will then be sent to your general practitioner. However, if there are some things that are very personal that you do not want disclosed at this time then you must discuss this with the psychiatrist. Some people ask that their family doctor not be informed about the consultation but this is not usually recommended, especially if they have referred you.

* * *

I hope that your visit to the psychiatrist will be a positive experience, since establishing trust and confidence in them as well as liking the doctor you meet is vital for recovery. If the visit is upsetting or unsatisfactory in some significant way please tell your general practitioner, who may be able to address your concerns.

> **Useful Contact**
>
> Mental Health Association of Ireland
> Mensana House, 6 Adelaide Street, Dun Laoighre, Co. Dublin
> Tel. (01) 2841166

I have been feeling very anxious and afraid lately. It has reached the stage where I can no longer concentrate at my job and my work is suffering. I would like to get help but I am afraid that I will have to pay a lot of money to see a counsellor/psychiatrist, which I cannot afford. What options do I have?

I am sorry that you are feeling under the weather at present. The first thing to do is to go to see your general practitioner. If you have a medical card then you will not have to pay for that consultation. It is possible that you will not need any further help if your doctor finds out the exact cause of your feelings of anxiety and so on. It may be necessary to rule out physical causes for this, so a simple blood test might be ordered.

Getting Help

If your general practitioner is unable to find a cause or make a definite diagnosis they may want to refer you for further evaluation by a psychiatrist or psychologist. Even if they do make a diagnosis they might still consider it best to refer you to a mental health professional for further treatment.

Whether you will be referred to a psychologist or psychiatrist will depend very much on your doctor's perception of your difficulties and your specific diagnosis. You would be entitled to the free services of a psychiatrist and the person to whom you would be referred would be determined by where you live, as these services are organised on an area basis.

A letter of referral would be sent and you would probably have to wait for an appointment. If your situation was deemed to be urgent, then you could be seen immediately. This would only be necessary if you were suicidal, acutely disturbed in your behaviour or unable to function at work and the initial emergency assessment would be made by the psychiatric registrar on call in the accident and emergency department.

Further Therapy

Once the psychiatrist has assessed you either in the out-patient clinic or as an emergency in the accident department you might then be referred onward to a psychologist or counsellor if a talking treatment were necessary. For example, if your problem was found to be due to alcohol abuse you would be referred to the substance abuse counsellors or if due to marital problems to a family therapist. These would all be available to you within the psychiatric services through your medical card, if you have one, so you may not have to pay.

Private Treatment

If your general practitioner wanted to refer you directly to a psychologist or counsellor rather than going through a psychiatrist initially this would have to be done privately and I understand you do not feel you could afford this. However, it would be worthwhile checking the cost of each visit, since the charge varies from therapist to therapist. Similarly, if you decide that you want to see a psychiatrist privately rather than going through the public system then you should also check the fee, as it may not be as high as you anticipate. If you have private health insurance this will cover the cost of seeing a psychiatrist (but not a psychologist) privately once it exceeds a certain amount.

Whether you opt to see a psychiatrist in the private or in the public sector you can be absolutely assured that they are all appropriately trained, as doctors initially and then in psychiatry, having taken two post-graduate examinations to achieve the necessary qualifications.

Communication

Whether you were seeing a psychologist or psychiatrist in the public or in the private system you would need to be referred by your doctor. In exceptional circumstances self-referral may be acceptable. Your doctor would also receive information about diagnosis and treatment following your visits and it would be considered best practice for your psychiatrist to interview a family member also in order to get objective information about your problems and the impact this is having on your life.

* * *

I advise you to discuss all the treatment options with your doctor. I hope you feel well soon.

Useful Contact

Mental Health Association of Ireland
Mensana House, 6 Adelaide Street, Dun Laoighre, Co. Dublin
Tel. (01) 2841166

My brother has recently come from the country to live near me. He has manic-depression and I want him to have a psychiatrist locally. However, he has been told by his doctor that the address we live in would not allow him to see the psychiatrist of his choice and we must see the designated one instead. This seems very rigid and both of us would now prefer that he saw a private psychiatrist based in a general hospital. What can I do?

You are right; this system seems very rigid and can be bureaucratic at times. However, since psychiatric hospitals were first established in Ireland, this has been the approach. In fact, throughout the world psychiatric services are organised in this way. Each hospital or unit covers a particular geographic area, known as a catchment area, and most are now broken down into even smaller units called sectors. The patient is therefore referred to the sector consultant and for this reason the exact location of where he lives is important.

Disadvantages

One of the problems with this type of sectorised service is that it does not allow the flexibility that you and your brother might wish for and there is little choice. The most serious difficulty is likely to arise if your brother and the psychiatrist do not get on well. In the event that they do not form a satisfactory relationship then you should write to the doctor who has overall charge of the local service, known as the Clinical Director. If you or your brother explains the situation alternative arrangements could possibly be made. This will be discretionary but all Clinical Directors would be very aware of the importance of a good therapeutic relationship with the treating doctor and hopefully would make appropriate provision for a change.

Rationale

The reason for the organisation of the psychiatric services in this way is to ensure equity in the responsibility for treatment and this is enshrined in the mental health legislation. This means that if for some reason a doctor covering a particular area refuses to treat a patient living there, then there is a breech of the duty and a complaint can be made to the Inspector of Mental Hospitals, who has responsibility for the proper discharge of these services. An investigation would then be conducted into the circumstances. A further advantage is that all the personnel that will be involved in the treatment of an individual patient should be available in that sector, in theory at any rate. These include community nurses, clinical psychologists, counsellors, occupational therapists, day hospitals and in-patient units as well as providing additional services such as psychotherapy and substance abuse services.

The other reason for setting geographic boundaries is so that specific services can be developed on an area basis and therefore be available in close proximity to where the patient lives.

Private Treatment

Those opting for private treatment can choose which psychiatrist to attend and this allows for greater choice and flexibility. However, a referral letter from the general practitioner would also be required as with the public clinics, but as there are very few private psychiatric units/hospitals available your brother might have to travel some distance. The private psychiatric hospitals offer very high quality treatment but should your brother need the services of a community nurse or other aftercare help then these would only be available through the sector team in the public service from whom he was already receiving treatment. This might be a problem for him if he needed significant input into his rehabilitation or if his illness became unstable and he needed to avail of day-hospital treatment. If your brother does decide to see a psychiatrist privately he should check if these ancillary services are available privately. It is important to realise that he cannot attend one psychiatrist for one aspect of his treatment and another for a different part, as the totality and continuity would be jeopardised.

* * *

I suggest that your brother discuss the options with his general practitioner, since they depend largely on his present psychiatric needs coupled with his preferences.

Useful Contact

Inspector of Mental Hospitals, Dept. of Health and Children, Hawkins House, Dublin 2, Tel. (01) 6354000

I have been attending my family doctor with panic attacks. I do not want anybody to know as some of my problems are very personal but I am worried that word might get out, as my doctor is friendly with my sister-in-law who is a nurse. What can I do about this?

You are probably aware that doctors are bound by confidentiality and in my experience they adhere very strictly to this principle. So even if your sister-in-law is friendly with your doctor, it is extremely unlikely that they are talking about your difficulties. In fact, the Medical Council, which governs the conduct of doctors in Ireland, states in its ethical guide that breaking confidentiality could lead to a charge of professional misconduct being brought against the doctor with very serious consequences for the doctor in question.

Confidentiality

In certain extenuating circumstances a doctor is allowed to disclose information and these are very specific. The first is when instructed by a court of law. For example, if a doctor was giving evidence in a court case involving the patient, if asked they would have to tell the truth even if the information disclosed was unpleasant or personal. The second is if a patient's life is at risk; then the doctor can also break a confidence so as to obtain help. For example, if the person indicated that suicide was being contemplated then the doctor could disclose this to another doctor or relevant person in order to save life. Similar rules apply with disclosures of murder or of serious criminal offences. However, if, as in your case there are no concerns of this nature, then you can be assured that information about you will not be divulged.

Gossiping

I understand your concern that your doctor might be talking with your sister-in-law about you but believe me doctors do not talk about specific named patients among each other or among friends because of the strict adherence to confidentiality. This caution extends even to the patient's case records. Suppose you were my patient and I wanted to get access to your notes from another doctor in the hospital then I would have to get your written permission to do so.

Even if you had a problem that was, for example, causing serious problems in your marriage such as having been abused in childhood, your doctor still could not explain the cause of your problems to your husband without your permission. Sometimes a doctor will ask to speak with a spouse, but this will be either for a therapy session or to obtain background information about the person's personality, symptoms and to assess the impact the problem is having on those in daily contact with the patient. Even in those circumstances it would still be inappropriate to disclose any information without explicit permission.

Breaching Confidence

If confidentiality is broken you could make a formal complaint to the Medical Council of Ireland, the body that regulates the conduct of doctors. They would carry out an investigation and if there were a suggestion, at face value, that this had happened then a full sworn inquiry would take place. This would involve you giving evidence, as in a court of law. The doctor would also be able to present their side and both of you could summon witnesses. If the doctor was found guilty of having broken confidentiality then one of the possible sanctions that could be applied to the doctor would be to prevent him from practising medicine by striking him off the medical register.

* * *

The medical profession in Ireland, as elsewhere, takes the requirement for confidentiality very seriously and you have nothing to fear. I suggest, however, that you openly discuss your concerns with your doctor.

Useful Contact

The Medical Council of Ireland
Lynn House, Lower Rathmines Road, Dublin 6, Tel. (01) 4983100

Psychological Therapies

All cases are unique, and very similar to others.

T.S. Eliot,
The Cocktail Party, *1949*

Psychological Therapies

My best friend has just started studying a course in counselling and every time we meet she talks jargon. She tells me that I have unconscious fears and that my superego is too punitive. What do these terms mean and what do they have to do with day-to-day life? She's driving me mad and at this rate our friendship will end.

I can sympathise with your exasperation at the change in your friend. This is often a feature when people begin to study or get interested in any of these psychological/psychiatric subjects. Students become inappropriately self-analytical and apply these theories to themselves and others.

The Unconscious

The terms that your friend is using are derived from a type of talking treatment known as psychoanalysis. It was developed by Freud towards the end of the 19th century as a result of treating women with unexplained physical symptoms. He concluded that there were psychological factors at work that explained these symptoms but that these were not known to the patient in her day-to-day thinking and functioning. This awareness of thoughts and events he called the conscious mind. The next level he called the pre-conscious, referring to thoughts and feelings that are easily available to consciousness – unpleasant events that have been deliberately pushed to the back of the mind fall into this category. The third level, the unconscious, describes thoughts, feelings and so on that are not available to conscious awareness without overcoming strong psychological resistance, known as defences.

Some people erroneously think of these as actual anatomical locations in the brain, but they are nothing more than shorthand for understanding how we deal psychologically with difficult emotions and thoughts; in other words, theories rather than physical realities. In using the language that she does, your friend is suggesting that you have fears about something that you have locked away in your mind without knowing it yourself and that manifests itself in other ways, perhaps in your personality or in some symptoms that you have.

The Superego

You say that your friend refers to the superego. Freud described the mind as having three functional parts – the *ego*, or the day-to-day manifestation of our personality, the superego, or conscience; the *id*, representing primitive impulses usually of a sexual nature; and the *superego*, acting as a kind of brake on the dangerous drives of the id resulting in the ego. In everyday language we often speak of somebody having a large ego, i.e. showing super-confidence.

Defences

Freud described various defences that the ego used to keep upsetting material from consciousness so that day-to-day functioning could continue. The best known is denial and you may have heard of people being described as "in denial". This means that events that happened are denied as ever having occurred, for example setting a table for a loved one even though that person has died. Unfortunately, the term is usually used incorrectly, described as the deliberate refusal to accept that an event has occurred. Denial is unconscious and therefore the person is unaware of the psychological trick they are playing on themselves.

Repression

Repression is also a well-known defence mechanism and it has attracted a lot of attention recently. It is a term that was used by Freud to explain why some memories that are painful cannot be recalled. He believed its purpose was to protect the person emotionally so that day-to-day functioning could continue. It is used nowadays to explain why memories of childhood abuse are often not recalled. Research to date shows that far from forgetting about the past, these upsetting events are all too easily remembered and although repression may occur it probably does not occur on the scale that was hitherto believed. What many people do is actively avoid thinking about certain things; this is not repression but is often confused with it.

Technique

The method of psychoanalysis involves reclining on a couch, with the analyst seated behind the patient. The aim is to encourage the free articulation of thoughts, fantasies and emotions, known as free association, with few verbal interventions from the analyst except to interpret the patient's associations.

Psychoanalysis is rarely used in everyday psychiatric or psychological practice as it is very time-consuming, requiring several sessions per week. The theories have spawned a whole approach to understanding psychological problems that is very useful in clinical practice and has attracted a lot of public interest. However, research into the merits of these theories and into the treatment method itself is lacking.

* * *

You should put up with your friend's self-indulgence for the moment, since, in a few months at most, it will pass and the knowledge that she is acquiring will come to rest more easily with her usual approach to life.

Useful Reading

Storr, Anthony (2001) *Freud: A Very Short Introduction*, Oxford University Press: Oxford

Useful Website

www.apsa.org/pubinfo/about.htm

My general practitioner has recently prescribed antidepressants for me as he has diagnosed depression. I do not mind taking medication in the short term but I would also like to have some "talking therapy". I want to use some therapy that works – what about counselling? Is it the same as cognitive therapy?

Cognitive therapy is a form of talking therapy that has been available since the 1980s. Psychologist Aaron Beck at the University of Pennsylvania first developed it.

Cognitions

Cognitive refers to our thoughts and perceptions about things around us. The basic premise is that our feelings, thoughts and behaviour are interlinked. In depression, the feelings or emotions are negative. These in turn give rise to negative thoughts as well as a failure to identify any positive things in life in the present, the past or the future. Therefore, the individual becomes hopeless. This negativity in turn affects behaviour so that instead of going out to meet friends the person withdraws into their own world; rather than going for a walk the person goes to bed to escape the painful thoughts and feelings. This model that links feelings, thoughts and behaviour can also be applied to anxiety disorders and even to specific emotions such as anger, embarrassment or shyness.

Techniques

Since the theory behind cognitive therapy can be applied to many common emotions, this treatment is used for many conditions besides depressive illness such as you have. These include panic disorder, social anxiety (extreme shyness), anger problems and deliberate self-harm.

Therapy is usually on a one-on-one basis but this may vary – for problems of shyness it is frequently conducted in a group setting. In general, several sessions are required before a response is noticed. In cognitive therapy the patient/client is actively involved in their treatment and the focus is on the present rather than on past traumas or on childhood. In this way, it differs significantly from other talking therapies. A daily diary is kept and emotions as well as the automatic thoughts that are generated are recorded. This task can be difficult initially, since people often confuse feelings and thoughts, but the task is easily learned. Using this approach the connection between the two can be clearly seen.

As treatment progresses the individual is taught to "talk back" to the negative thoughts – in other words more helpful and alternative responses to the thoughts are written down. Thus, the person with depression or anxiety learns to challenge the automatic negative thoughts that occur and so the cycle of negative thoughts worsening the depression or anxiety is broken.

A further strategy in cognitive therapy is to examine tasks in a piecemeal fashion. All of us when overwhelmed with work or personal problems see the totality of what confronts us rather than taking each problem at a time and drawing up a priority list. Using this simple strategy the magnitude of the problems seems more manageable.

Trained Therapist

A trained cognitive therapist must deliver cognitive therapy as it is highly specialised. Many people who describe themselves as therapists, although trained in other talking treatments, may not necessarily be skilled in cognitive therapy and so you must check this before you begin. Most clinical psychologists have such training but you should not take it for granted.

Counselling

Finally, you ask if cognitive therapy is the same as counselling. The problem is that the term "counselling" is used by most people to describe any form of treatment that does not involve medication. However, professionals describe counselling as one form of non-drug treatment, since there are numerous approaches to talking with and listening to those who have emotional or personal problems. The public and professionals therefore see counselling differently from each other and this can cause great confusion. In counselling, the focus is on the expression of emotion and on the exploration of the problem. Listening by the therapist is central but advice is not offered, since a central tenet of counselling is that it must be non-directive and the client/patient must make the decisions.

* * *

Cognitive therapy has been shown to be effective in the treatment of depressive illness both when it is initially diagnosed and as an aid to preventing relapse. In combination with medication it has been shown to be better than either treatment alone. You are right to consider this therapy and I wish you well.

Useful Reading

Bates, Tony (1999) *Depression: The Common Sense Approach*, New Leaf (an imprint of Gill and McMillan Ltd): Dublin

Useful Website

www.rcpsych.ac.uk/info/factsheets/pfaccog.htm

Psychosexual Disorders

Sexual problems have disappeared in the 21st century.

Common myth

I am thirty and for the past twelve years I get irritable, tense, depressed and hopeless before my period. I also feel out of control. My family tell me that I am a changed person during that phase and that I am impossible to live with. I have lost several boyfriends as a result. My doctor has been treating me and gave me the "pill", but without any benefit. She now wants me to see a psychiatrist – but I'm not crazy. What should I do? I have heard that a high-fibre diet might help.

I can understand why you are surprised at the suggestion that you should see a psychiatrist for what appears to be a gynaecological problem. To some extent you are right, but you may have some psychological symptoms that would benefit from brief psychiatric help. Most people who attend psychiatrists are not "crazy" but just have some emotional problem that requires extra help.

Physical and Psychological

The usual features of premenstrual syndrome, PMS as it is now called, are a mixture of mainly physical symptoms, such as weight gain, feeling bloated and tiredness, with some emotional symptoms also, particularly tension and depression. Feelings of being out of control are common in this disorder too. Most of the current treatments such as the "pill" and water tablets (diuretics) to reduce the bloated feeling only help the physical symptoms. For this reason, the psychological symptoms require additional treatment and your general practitioner may be able to tailor her treatment once she has received a report from a psychiatrist.

Diary

One of the first things you should do is keep a diary of your moods over several months. If your mood changes are due to PMS you will see a clear drop in your spirits immediately before menstruation that lifts within a few days of it beginning. There should be no other change in mood during the cycle until the next cycle, again at the same time, with the pattern repeating over several months.

Many women attribute low mood to their cycle even when there is no connection and this will only emerge when you keep a diary. Often those who think they have PMS are in fact suffering with depressive disorders that are exacerbated during the pre-menstrual phase. This is a common problem. Additional symptoms would then be present, including sleep and appetite disturbance, panic attacks and poor concentration.

Caution

There has been a lot of publicity about alternative treatments for PMS including vitamins, aerobic exercise, reducing caffeine intake, relaxation exercises and high-fibre diets. Many of these are of unproven efficacy but remain popular for mild symptoms. Low salt diets are useful only when symptoms due to fluid retention are prominent. Oral contraceptives do not help the psychological symptoms – and may even worsen them.

The main treatment for the psychological symptoms is with antidepressants, known as the SSRIs. About five such preparations are available and they work at very low doses, much lower than those used in depression. Also, unlike the response in depression, which takes several weeks, when used in PMS a response is shown within a few days and you may only need to take them for a couple of weeks of each cycle while the symptoms are prominent. After a trial of treatment for about one year the need for medication can be re-evaluated.

* * *

The main benefit from seeing a psychiatrist is to be certain that you have PMS and not depressive illness. In addition, if there are major family problems as a result of your condition then help with restoring relationships will also be available. If you have PMS you will not need to see a psychiatrist for more than a few visits. You should follow your general practitioner's advice.

Useful Website

www.pms.org.uk

I am fifty and my doctor tells me I am going through the menopause. I am feeling a bit low in my spirits too and I would like to go on HRT. I am also worried that I may become like my aunt, who was hospitalised after a nervous breakdown during the menopause and remained there for several years.

There are many myths about the menopause, the most common being that women are more prone to major mental health problems at this time. There is little evidence to support this and studies have found that depressive illness, schizophrenia and manic-depression are not especially common at this time of life. Indeed, these disorders are more common during the earlier years of life and for many women the menopause is associated with a greater sense of well-being than previously.

It is true that some women who have depressive episodes exclusively associated with childbirth and not at any other time of life may be at an increased risk of depression in the pre-menopausal years. If you have never been depressed before it is highly unlikely that you would now have a hormone-related depression.

Coincidence

It is also important to bear in mind that the risk of depression is life-long and so if you have a depressive illness now it is likely to be coincidental. Your doctor will be able to tell you if you have a clinical depression now and if you have then you are unlikely to benefit from HRT.

In particular, symptoms such as tearfulness, poor concentration, feelings of tension and irritability would suggest a depressive illness. There have been many studies examining the effects of HRT in those who develop depressive illness during the menopause and there is no evidence that hormone replacement is useful in treating this when compared to placebo, though it may help the menopausal symptoms such as hot flushes. However, antidepressants have been shown to be significantly helpful in treating depression at this time of life.

During the menopause some women feel a little below par, although they are not clinically depressed. In these women HRT is effective like a mental tonic and this is determined by the amount of oestrogen rather than progesterone. Your doctor should choose the preparation with this in mind.

Myths

Another received wisdom is that women become odd and strange during the menopause – again there is absolutely nothing in the scientific research to suggest that mental health problems of this magnitude are especially related to hormone changes at this time. It sounds as though your aunt had a serious mental illness and it was almost certainly coincidental rather than caused by the menopause. You do not need to be worried about this happening to you.

People often speak of the "empty nest" syndrome. This is not a psychiatric disorder but a manifestation of the understandable sense of loss that mothers and sometimes fathers feel when children leave home and the bustle of everyday life slows and becomes more sedate. Very occasionally, this can lead to a depression, rather like being bereaved, but usually there is a successful adaptation to the change even though it may be lonely initially.

Male Menopause

There has been some discussion about the possibility of a male menopause but none of the physiological changes that happen to women have been described in men. Instead, as some men approach middle life they begin to question what their hard work has achieved, particularly if they have neglected other areas such as their family or their intellectual, spiritual or emotional side and this leads to questions such as "Where am I going?", "What have I achieved?" and "Who am I?" Such self-scrutiny may not be abnormal and may lead to positive changes in outlook and behaviour.

* * *

Essentially your general practitioner will tell you if you are depressed. If you are not, HRT may boost your sense of well-being. So forget old wives' tales about the horrors of the "change"; you are no more likely to suffer doleful moods and unpredictable rages caricatured in the popular press at this time of life than at any other.

Useful Website

www.bcrmh.com/disorders/menopause.htm

Psychosexual Disorders

My sixteen-year-old son recently told me that he thought he might be gay. I was surprised, as I had always thought he was interested in girls. I know he has many male friends but I never suspected anything like this. He is not effeminate at all and is interested in the usual things that most boys are, such as sport and rock music. I know very little about homosexuality and I don't know what to do.

I am sure you were surprised to hear this from your son, but it is a credit to you and to his relationship with you that he can discuss such matters. Being able to confide in one's family is the best protection against major emotional problems, whatever one's sexuality.

Curiosity

Many boys during this phase of their sexual development are uncertain about their sexual orientation and his comment to you may be simply a reflection of this uncertainty. However, most homosexual men report being attracted to their own sex from a young age, often in childhood. That is not to say that any sexual activity occurred at that time, merely a feeling of being different to other boys and of a lack of interest in girls. Some homosexual men also report relationships with women prior to their acceptance of their sexual orientation. This probably comes from a wish, in some teenagers, to be heterosexual, while in others it may be an expression of uncertainty about their true orientation.

Myths

There are several myths about being gay and one is that homosexual men are effeminate. This is incorrect and although some do display effeminate behaviours and traits, many others do not. Another myth is that homosexuality is a psychiatric disorder that can be cured. This is also untrue: since 1973 it has not been viewed as an illness within the profession, as it is not especially associated with any impairment in day-to-day functioning and any distress associated with it stems from not accepting one's sexual orientation or from the attitude of others to it. It is important to realise that homosexuality does not appear to be a matter of choice.

Contentment

Many mothers are upset when they hear that a son is gay and above all fear for his ultimate happiness. However, there is no reason why a homosexual man should not live a fulfilling and successful life. Therefore, if your son is gay, provided he has support, his life should not be marred, unless he has difficulty accepting his orientation or others react negatively.

Causes

The early studies of the frequency of homosexuality suggested a prevalence of 10 per cent in the general population. Recent studies have significantly lowered this figure and a 1993 study in the US found that 1 per cent of men reported being exclusively homosexual and 2 per cent reported a life history of homosexual experiences. As with all studies of sexual activity, the possibility that the findings are unreliable cannot be discounted due to either bravado or reticence on the part of those being interviewed.

Various psychological theories have explored the reasons for homosexual orientation, including lack of effective fathering, a strong fixation on the mother and stunting of masculine development by the parents. Other possibilities have included low levels of circulating sex hormones or exposure to low levels of male hormones during foetal development. However, these theories are speculative and have *not* been proven: some studies have corroborated them; others have not. There was great controversy a few years ago when some researchers suggested a genetic basis for sexual orientation, but no specific chromosome has been identified. As yet, no single cause has been definitively identified.

* * *

Your son is only just beginning to express his sexuality and there is no way of knowing what his ultimate orientation will be. However, you should remain open to discussing this with him without intruding upon his own doubts at present. You might also suggest he discuss his uncertainty with a professional if his doubts continue.

Useful Reading

Farber, M. (1995) *Human Sexuality*, Macmillan: New York

Useful Contact

MRCS (Marriage and Relationship Counselling Services)
Tel. (01) 6799341

Psychosexual Disorders

I am very embarrassed by my problem. I am sixty-two years old and I have a successful business. My marriage is very good but recently I have become impotent. I just cannot hold an erection and I am so embarrassed. Thankfully, my wife is wonderful and she says it does not bother her. She wants me to go to my doctor but I am shy of this, as we play golf together. Perhaps it is just the effect of getting older. Can you help?

Your wife is correct. You must visit your doctor; if you are embarrassed then you should see a doctor that you do not know as well. It might be time to go for a general health check anyway. Some hospitals now run whole-day assessments and screen for a number of common disorders. This would provide you with the opportunity to discuss your problem with a doctor who is a stranger to you. One of the many myths about impotence is that it is a consequence of ageing. While older men may take longer to arouse, impotence, now usually termed erectile dysfunction (ED), is not due to increasing age.

Common Disorder

The first thing to remember is that ED is common and 15–25 per cent of 65-year-old men experience it. I suggest that you be frank with your doctor, since he will undoubtedly have seen many others with the same problem. Your doctor will ask about the effect it is having on your marriage. They will also ask questions about the quality of your relationship in general, as marital difficulties can contribute to this problem. You should tell your doctor if you are having any other physical symptoms, since there are a number of physical and psychological conditions that can cause erectile problems. Finally, remember to take a list of any medications that you are taking, including herbal remedies, with you to the consultation.

Physical Problems

Diabetes is probably one of the most common illnesses causing ED. Abnormalities in hormone-producing glands such as the thyroid can also cause ED and must be considered. When the arteries are getting hard and narrow due to arteriosclerosis impotence can develop. It can sometimes follow surgery for prostate problems. Some neurological conditions that effect sensation might cause impotence also. Depression is a common cause of ED and the treatments used in depression may themselves contribute. You did not mention if you drink a lot of alcohol; alcohol is commonly associated with ED, as is recreational drug use in younger people. If you are taking tablets for high blood pressure you might also be at risk. Finally, any anxiety associated with the condition might be adding to the problem, even if there is a physical cause.

Investigations

It is unlikely that you will have to go to hospital, although of course this ultimately depends on what the initial out-patient examination and investigations reveal. Your doctor will carry out an examination of your heart and blood vessels to check for arteriosclerosis (narrowing). In addition, you will be given a neurological examination. This will take just a few minutes. You may then have to give a sample of urine and have some blood tests.

Treatment

The success of treatment depends on the cause. If it is due to diabetes or one of the hormonal disorders when that is brought under control the ED should improve. If it is due to excessive alcohol, cutting down your intake can improve the condition, as can treating depression if that is responsible. "Viagra" may be helpful, especially if the problem does not resolve fully, although if you have angina you cannot take it as it may interact with treatment for this condition.

* * *

The most important thing to remember is that ED is treatable in all age groups and it is essential that you get medical help sooner rather than later.

Useful Website

www.impotence.org

Useful Contact

The Impotence Association
www.impotence.org.uk
Tel. (0044) 20 8767 7791

Psychosexual Disorders

I am a thirty-year-old woman with an embarrassing problem. I cannot have sexual intercourse as I find it very painful. My husband and I have not yet consummated our recent marriage. The thought of sex really puts me off. Somebody suggested I might consider "Viagra". What do you think?

I am sorry that you are experiencing this problem and it must be very distressing for you and your husband that you have not consummated your marriage. You certainly must seek professional help for this. Believe it or not, sexual problems of this type are not all that uncommon – up to 15 per cent of women have some sexual problem during their lifetime. So you are not alone.

Viagra

I would not recommend Viagra in these circumstances. Even though a few studies have found it helpful in women who have low sexual interest, it is not licensed for this purpose and recent research has found it to be unhelpful. The reasons for this are simple. In men it acts to increase blood flow to the penis and in this way facilitates sexual arousal. In women, however, sexual response is much more psychological in origin and it will be impaired if the woman is tired or stressed, on certain medications, has low interest or has specific conditions such as vaginismus. It does not have any effect on pain during intercourse and does not increase sexual interest.

Pain

The pain that you describe is termed dyspareunia (pronounced dis-pa-roon-ia) and has many causes. In a young adult such as you, it may be caused by not being adequately aroused. For example, if you are tense or if the technique your husband uses is unsatisfactory then you will not become excited enough and this will cause pain. If you have an infection such as thrush or if you are on certain medications such as antidepressants then the lining of the vagina will be dry and this might also cause discomfort when intercourse is attempted. Uterine problems such as endometriosis might also cause pain or you may be allergic to some of the hygiene products that you use.

Interest

It is not clear from your letter if your lack of interest in sex has been of long standing or if it has developed secondary to the discomfort that you experience.

Your doctor would need to establish this in the first instance and if the pain you experience is secondary to your low interest then the treatment would be very different from a primary pain disorder. One of the common reasons for loss of libido (sexual interest) is anxiety, tiredness or depression and these would need to be ruled out also.

What is your attitude to sex? Does the thought of it repel you? Have you had bad prior sexual experiences? For instance, if there is any possibility that you were ever sexually abused or assaulted you might understandably find sexual activity difficult and painful due to low arousal levels stemming from these traumas.

Vaginismus

One of the most common reasons for difficulty with intercourse is vaginismus, a condition in which the muscles of the vagina contract involuntarily. The result is an inability to have intercourse and pain is experienced during attempts. This is natures' way of protecting the vagina from anticipated pain and sometimes it occurs even when the doctor attempts a genital examination. If this is the cause then it is very treatable, with an 80 per cent success rate.

Treatment

It is essential that you and your husband go to a therapist trained in sexual problems. You should both attend together, since this problem is affecting both of you. A detailed sexual history will be taken from you separately and, of course, what each of you discloses will be confidential.

* * *

I hope it all works out for you both and the first step is asking for help, as you have done.

Useful Reading

Stone, R. (1998) *Understanding Sex and Relationships*, Sheldon: London

Useful Website

www.sexwithoutpain.com/dyspareunia.htm

Useful Contact

MRCS (Marriage and Relationship Counselling Services)
Tel. (01) 6799341

I am nineteen years old and I have been feeling very upset for the past few months. The reason is that a distant relative abused me sexually when I was ten years old. I thought I would be able to forget about it. Unfortunately, this did not happen and in my college course we have recently been covering sexual abuse. This upset me and I plucked up the courage to tell my parents. They are devastated and want me to go for counselling. I am frightened that talking about it will be too embarrassing and that I will get even more depressed. I am at college and I don't want anything to interfere with that.

You did the correct thing in telling your parents about the awful trauma that you have had to go through. Their support is vital to your healing from this and they are quite right – you should seek help as soon as you feel ready. It is tempting to think that you will be able to put the abuse to the back of your mind without professional help or that you will be able to delay it. However, in reality this is not going to be possible, especially since you are already distressed and understandably upset about what has happened and it is very much on your mind.

Depression

One of the risks of not seeking any professional help is that the distress you are experiencing now will continue and may even increase as time passes. Sometimes this can result in full-blown clinical depression and at that point you may need therapy anyway. Depression that occurs against a background of sexual abuse can be very difficult to treat, so it is best to avoid this developing at all.

Positive Aspects

You are fortunate that your parents are so supportive. This in itself will make it easier for you to face therapy. It will also make a successful emotional outcome for you more likely. A further positive aspect is the fact that you seem to be getting on with your education rather than buckling under the weight of what has happened in the past. It is also very helpful that you realise the relevance of the abuse to your present mood state.

Therapy

A therapist will work at your pace and if there are times when you feel unable to talk about the past, then your need for this silence will be respected. Many people find it very difficult to talk about what has happened, at least initially, and sometimes it is helpful to put in writing your story and your narrative of those events. This may make talking easier.

When you begin therapy, check how many sessions and over what period you will be attending. Since you are positive in outlook about the future and as your parents are fully behind you, therapy may be completed within one year, although, of course, there is much individual variation also. You do not indicate the exact nature of the abuse that you suffered but the more severe and persistent the abuse the longer the duration of therapy.

There is no reason to think that therapy might interfere with your career, although if you become distressed your concentration may be affected, at least in the short term. It is during these periods that some people request longer gaps between appointments although this should be avoided if possible, since it prolongs the whole treatment process. You should not run away from what has happened to you or let it control you; you should face it and resolve your feelings about it and about the abuser.

* * *

Therapy will consist of you ventilating your thoughts and feelings about what has happened, in particular your feelings of self-blame, sadness, dirt and anger at these events. Ultimately, you will be helped to move on from the past and to look to the positive future that you have. You would be unwise to carry the burden of the abuse yourself, so you should follow your parents' advice when you feel ready.

Useful Reading

Kinnerely, H. (2000) *Overcoming Childhood Trauma*, London: Constable and Robinson

Useful Website

www.musc.edu/cvc/
(Open file then click on Child Physical and Sexual Abuse: Treatment Guidelines)

Useful Contact

Laragh, Prospect House, Prospect Road, Glasnevin, Dublin 9, Tel. (01) 8335044
(Counselling service for victims of sexual abuse established by the Eastern Regional Health Authority)

I was sexually abused as a child and I thought I had dealt with it. I am twenty-eight and I have never had any problems until recently, when all the publicity about sexual abuse has upset me. I am now feeling depressed and my doctor wants me to take antidepressants and go for counselling. I just don't know what to do, as I am scared of talking to others about what happened.

From what you say, it is clear that you have not dealt with abuse. If you had, you would not be so upset and I am sure your general practitioner would not be suggesting medication. You should seriously consider going for counselling about it.

Therapists

It is important that you find a suitable therapist – this means finding somebody with the right expertise. This may be a psychiatrist or a psychologist. Other options are the counsellors in the Rape Crisis Centres, but there are likely to be long waiting lists before you can commence therapy. Some health boards have established services dedicated to counselling those who have been sexually abused. Whichever professional you opt for, therapy is almost certain to be one to one, so feeling comfortable with your therapist is very important also. I can understand why you would not want to speak about such personal matters in front of others so you should check with your therapist what is envisaged, in particular if your therapy will be individual or in a group. I do not think it appropriate that in the early stages of therapy you should have to disclose personal matters to strangers and I believe most professionals would sympathise with this view.

Medication

Taking medication is no barrier to having counselling and most therapists would agree with this. Sometimes medication is helpful to those who have been abused and are displaying significant depression such that day-to-day functioning is affected. I am unsure if your depression is affecting you in this way. However, in my experience antidepressants are not always helpful and the improvement in mood often only takes place as therapy progresses and as the person comes to terms with what has happened.

Beginning Therapy

Anticipating what therapy might be like is the most worrying for most people. Therapists differ in their approach. The sessions, usually about an hour long, consist of you speaking about whatever you wish to bring up. Nothing will be imposed and if you just want to sit quietly because it is too upsetting to talk about the past then that is acceptable. Sometimes it is helpful to write about what has happened and if you find talking difficult, then your therapist may suggest this as a way of breaking the barrier.

An issue that may arise later is whether this matter will have to be reported to the gardaí. It is impossible for me to answer this now. However, if the person who abused you still has contact with children then your therapist will be obliged to report it. If the person does not, perhaps they are elderly and in a home, then there may be some discretion exercised, but that depends on the organisation that is providing your therapy. You should clarify this at the first session so as to avoid later misunderstanding.

Duration of Therapy

The duration of therapy varies – it will depend on how you deal with the trauma. Some people become very upset and distressed and have to slow down the pace of therapy or even terminate it for a time. Others, although finding the process difficult, do continue with support. It is rarely of short duration unless the person has already come to terms with the abuse. You should think in terms of months or longer, depending on the extent of the abuse and the impact it has had on your life.

* * *

You must keep reminding yourself that therapy is necessary if you are to put the abuse behind you.

Useful Contact

Laragh, 7 Marne Villas, Dublin 7, Tel. (01) 8383323
(A counselling service for victims of sexual abuse established by the Eastern Regional Health Authority)

Schizophrenia

People with schizophrenia tend to be violent.

Common myth

What does it mean to be paranoid? My daughter often tells me that I am paranoid, especially when I question what she does – she is only sixteen. I was discussing this recently with my neighbour and she told me that an uncle of hers was diagnosed by a psychiatrist as being paranoid several years ago. Could I have a mental illness?

Unfortunately, the word "paranoid" is often used by those who do not understand what it means and it is most often incorrectly used to describe somebody who is overly concerned or pre-occupied with something. So your daughter might be using the term to mean that you are too concerned about her behaviour. That is not the correct meaning of the word. Its accurate usage is to describe feelings of suspicion or of being put upon by others. The person who believes that others are talking about them or are being critical of them when in fact they are not is said to be paranoid.

Psychiatric Diagnosis

Paranoid psychosis is a psychiatric disorder and your neighbour's uncle may have had this condition. It means that he was suspicious of others or of what they were saying or doing to him when he had no reason to be. However, for it to be diagnosed the degree of mistrust and suspiciousness must have been significant. For example, he may have believed that he was being talked about or that some person or organisation was persecuting him. Alternatively, he may have believed that there was a conspiracy against him or that his wife was having an affair when in fact she was not. In their mildest form, these thoughts can be argued away and the person can accept that they are getting things out of proportion but when they are very severe the thoughts remain fixed. In this severe form of paranoia, beliefs like these that are held with absolute conviction are known as delusions.

Causes of Paranoia

There a number of reasons why somebody such as your neighbour's uncle might come to hold paranoid beliefs that are false. Some people are born with a suspicious turn of mind and they see slights and insults everywhere. Usually, however, their life is not too badly affected and they work, form relationships and make some friends. They can also be reassured that their suspicions are false and represent an exaggeration. These people are said to have paranoid personalities. In some instances, drinking alcohol to excess can also make people suspicious and this is probably the most common cause, with concerns about the partner's fidelity being the most prominent. Drugs such as cocaine and amphetamines can also cause feelings of persecution and may even lead to violence against others who are believed to be causing the persecution.

There is also an illness known as paranoid schizophrenia in which these delusions of being persecuted are combined with hearing voices and having other unusual experiences. Sometimes those with diseases of the brain such as Alzheimer's disease or epilepsy may also become paranoid.

"Convince a Man against his Will"

The first thing to remember is that trying to convince somebody who holds these false beliefs with absolute conviction that they are mistaken can entrench them further. If the beliefs are fleeting and not so firmly held then it may be possible, temporarily at least, to curtail them. Of course, any substances such as illicit drugs or excessive alcohol intake should be controlled as that in itself may lead to a substantial improvement. Medication is necessary when the paranoid symptoms are due to a schizophrenic illness or to brain disease. If the person is paranoid about a spouse or other person living in the house with them, it may be necessary to separate them as a safety measure since violence can occasionally ensue.

Misusing the Term

It is highly likely that your daughter is misusing the word and that you do not have a psychiatric illness. However, when people are paranoid they often do not realise it and if you are in doubt then you should ask others in your family, taking care to explain what is meant by paranoia. Indeed, if you discuss it with your daughter she may well agree that she has been using the term inappropriately. Others would certainly notice if you were suspicious when there was no reason to be.

* * *

It is unfortunate that words such as "paranoid" are used so loosely, as it can cause a lot of confusion.

Useful Website
www.hoptechno.com/paranoia.htm

I recently overheard people at work describing me as a "schizophrenic". I was devastated by this and I confronted them. They told me, in no uncertain terms, that I was moody and difficult to work with and that at times they thought I might be violent. They also said that they thought I had a split personality and that I had schizophrenia. I am devastated by these assertions and wonder if indeed I do have schizophrenia.

I am sorry that your colleagues seem so negative about you. It may be helpful for you to discuss this issue with the human resources manager in order to clarify the perception that other people in your firm generally have of you. Perhaps these people have a personal grudge against you, in which case it is a matter that could be resolved with help from HR. Alternatively, it may be that you have some problems relating to colleagues at work, in which case you may need professional help from an occupational or clinical psychologist.

Schizophrenia

Unfortunately, schizophrenia is a term that is often used very loosely rather than in its true clinical meaning. Schizophrenia is a psychiatric illness that affects young people, usually. The main feature is loss of touch with reality in the form of hallucinations. These usually consist of hearing voices when there is nobody about or nothing to explain them. Delusions are another element of the loss of contact with reality. These are false beliefs that are out of context with the culture: for example, the person might believe that they are being spied on or that their actions are under the control of outside agencies. If the illness is untreated, a personality change occurs, resulting in increasing withdrawal, lack of motivation and an inability to hold any meaningful conversation.

It is clear that you certainly do not have this illness.

Split Personality

Regrettably, the term "split personality" is often used by the general public to describe schizophrenia. Schizophrenia most definitely is not split personality and the confusion arose because of the splitting of parts of mental function from reality, in the form of hallucinations and delusions. The term "schizophrenic" is often used in day-to-day conversation to describe having contradictory or ambivalent attitudes to a particular matter; this is an inappropriate use of the term.

Violence

There is a mistaken belief that those with schizophrenia are prone to violence. However, most people with schizophrenia are not violent, although occasionally during the very acute phase of the illness, before treatment commences, there may be agitation and anger. By far the most common cause of aggression is not any form of psychiatric illness but difficulty controlling impulsive behaviour associated with alcohol and illicit drug abuse. Perhaps you are quick tempered and fiery – this may be the real reason that they think you have the potential to be violent. Perhaps you should examine your alcohol intake and whether you use illegal drugs.

* * *

It is important that you discuss your predicament with your HR manager and then seek help if you feel you need it. You can do so in the knowledge that you do not have "split personality" or schizophrenia. The language your workmates use is both cruel and offensive to you. It is also inaccurate and stigmatising of those who suffer with schizophrenia.

Useful Reading

The Schizophrenia Handbook (2002), published by Schizophrenia Ireland

Useful Contact

Schizophrenia Ireland
38 Blessington Street, Dublin 7, Tel. (01) 8601620, e-mail: schizi@iol.ie

My brother has had schizophrenia for years although he is well at present. Over the years he has required admission to hospital on many occasions and I have seen him in a very disturbed state. I am worried that my son may inherit this illness. Can you give me any information on this?

Your concerns are understandable and there is no simple answer. What is definitely known is that it is uncertain if the presence of schizophrenia in a family member will definitely cause it in another relative. In other words, there is no 100 per cent certainty that your son will get this illness.

Genetic Studies

However, a wide range of genetic studies strongly suggest that there is a genetic component, so that a person is more likely to develop schizophrenia if other family members have it and that the risk increases as the genetic closeness of the relationship increases. First-degree relatives (children, siblings) of those with schizophrenia have a higher risk than second-degree relatives (cousins, nephews). An identical twin whose co-twin has schizophrenia has the highest risk and this applies even when the twins are separated at birth by adoption, proving that it is not just the common environment or rearing practices that are responsible. The size of the risk (also called concordance) increases from 8 per cent for a non-twin sibling to 12 per cent if one parent has schizophrenia and 40 per cent if both parents have schizophrenia. The highest concordance is for identical twins – 47 per cent of co-twins will develop the illness. In the case of your son, in the absence of any other information, it would seem that his risk is certainly less than 8 per cent.

In view of the increasing risk with increasing closeness of relationship there have been numerous studies attempting to identify the actual gene responsible. So far, it is clear that there is no single gene involved and abnormalities have been reported at four or five gene sites. Therefore, the inheritance of the illness in any one person cannot be predicted and so it cannot be predicted in your son.

Environmental Factors

Although genes determine the vulnerability to schizophrenia, it is recognised that external factors impinge upon this to trigger the illness. For example, the abuse of drugs such as amphetamines greatly increases the risk of becoming ill with schizophrenia and a recent study showed that heavy cannabis use (defined as "smoking" twice per week) increased the risk seven-fold.

Another finding that has generated a considerable amount of research is the finding that those who have schizophrenia are more likely to have been born in the early months of the year, between January and April. In the southern hemisphere the months of birth are more often between July and September. These findings suggest that some season-specific risk factors are operating, such as a virus or a seasonal dietary change.

Biological Changes

Recent research has focussed on the biological changes that occur in the brain of those with schizophrenia. The predominant view is that there is too much dopamine in certain areas of the brain and that when certain dopamine receptors (those parts of the nerve endings that dopamine stimulates) are abnormal, symptoms known as positive symptoms are to the fore; when other dopamine receptors are affected negative symptoms are prominent. With the advent of modern radiological techniques it is becoming possible to visualise which parts of the brain may be affected and the impact that medication is having on them. These studies suggest that in those who are not yet treated but have symptoms there are changes to the front part of the brain. This would seem to suggest that schizophrenia is a disease of the brain and a far cry from the older theory that mothers were to blame.

* * *

In light of the ongoing research and its tentative findings there is no need for you to worry that your parenting style may cause schizophrenia and I strongly advise you not to be overly watchful of your son.

Useful Reading

Mueser, K.T. and Gingrich, S. (1994) *Coping with Schizophrenia: A Guide for Families*, New Harbinger: Oakland, CA

Useful Website

www.priory.com/psych/neurodev.htm

Useful Contact

Schizophrenia Ireland
38 Blessington Street, Dublin 7, Tel. (01) 8601620, e-mail: schizi@iol.ie

Schizophrenia

My son has recently been diagnosed with schizophrenia. I am thrilled that he has responded well to treatment and he hopes to return to work soon. However, I am wracked with guilt as we never had a great relationship and I have been told by his doctor that this may cause him to relapse again unless things improve between us. Is this correct? I could not live with myself if I thought I had caused his illness.

I am delighted that your son is improving and returning to his usual routine. You should not torment yourself with the fear that you may have caused his illness as there is no scientific research to back up this view. As your doctors have told you there is some evidence that relapse may be related to poor family relationships, but help is available to remedy this.

Old Theories

Research into schizophrenia is relatively new and has come to prominence only in the past twenty years. Before that, when our understanding of the illness was limited, there were many suggestions as to what caused it. Some psychiatrists insisted that it was not an illness at all but a mark of "sanity" in an "insane world". Anybody having contact with sufferers would realise that such a view is nonsensical, seeing the suffering of those with schizophrenia, especially when they are untreated. This view also ignores the suicide rate among those with schizophrenia, which in past was about 10 per cent over a ten-year period. That figure should significantly diminish as better treatments are available and for a sizeable number, among them your son hopefully, the quality of life can be very good.

Blame

One of the theories from that time was that faulty communication between mother and child lead to this illness. The belief was that mothers gave simultaneously conflicting messages to their children, for example telling the child how much they were loved while looking angry. This became known as the "double bind theory" and held sway during the 1950s. The belief was that the child, unsure of how to respond, retreated into the world of schizophrenia. However, this has now been disproven.

Another fashionable theory from that period centred on divisions of power within the family, known as a family schism and skew. In one type of family there was a schism between the parents, with one getting overly close to the child of the opposite sex. In the other type of family there was a power struggle between the parents, with one becoming dominant. Both of these theories were nothing more than speculation and when they were subjected to scientific examination they were shown to have no foundation.

Unfortunately, these theories from time to time still receive credence in "pop" psychology/psychiatry in spite of the absence of anything to back them up. Among the mainstream of psychiatry and psychology they have long been discarded.

Emotion

In the early 1980s, researchers did find that those with schizophrenia living in families that were either hostile, critical or emotionally over-involved had a higher risk of relapse, even with medication, than those in the more usual type of family, i.e. one that was concerned and loving without being over-controlling. This pattern of interacting was termed "high expressed emotion" (high EE). The research also showed that if attempts were made to improve the family's understanding of the illness through family education then by reducing EE relapse lessened. Family therapy to help with the over-involvement and criticism had the same effect. However, research also found that if these interventions did not help, reducing the face-to-face contact between parents and child to less than 35 hours each week had the same effect. In other words, once the problem is identified, strategies can be put in place to correct its effects. Regrettably, some have mistakenly taken this to imply that certain types of family cause schizophrenia, whereas in fact this type of family is associated with relapse and is amenable to intervention.

***

You need have no guilt that you have in any way caused your son's illness; these theories that have suggested this are from the past and have caused untold sadness to many families. Please talk with your son's doctors to decide on the best approach to improving your relationship with your son and ultimately to keeping him well, as it seems to be relapses that his doctor is concerned about.

Useful Reading

Torrey, E.F. (2001) *Surviving Schizophrenia: A Manual for Families, Consumers and Providers*, Quill Publishers: Kolkata, India (Available from Schizophrenia Ireland)

Useful Contact

Schizophrenia Ireland
38 Blessington Street, Dublin 7, Tel. (01) 8601620, e-mail: schizi@iol.ie

A cousin of mine has schizophrenia and attends the psychiatric clinic regularly. He is well and able to work but still on medication. I think he should have counselling and I feel he doesn't need drugs any more. He tells me that his doctor disagrees.

There are indeed some psychiatric conditions, and schizophrenia is among them, where medication is the mainstay of treatment. This is not for any perverse reason but because when compared with other approaches, such as psychotherapy, it has been shown in research studies to be significantly more effective.

However, there are also psychiatric disorders less serious than schizophrenia, such as phobias, where medication has virtually no role and where the principal treatment is behavioural or some form of talking therapy. Eating disorders and substance addiction, whilst very serious, are largely treated using talking treatments, without the use of medication.

So the therapy depends on the condition from which the person suffers. In many instances both medication and some type of psychotherapy are combined.

Counselling or Psychotherapy

In everyday parlance the term counselling is used to describe any therapy that does not involve drugs. However, in the medical profession counselling is but one particular type of talking treatment along with a number of others, which combined are termed "the psychotherapies". For the purposes of answering your question I will use the term "counselling" as you do – to describe all the non-drug treatments that are available.

First Do No Harm

As doctors we have to treat our patients with proven techniques. Before they are released onto the market for use by the medical profession, all medications are subject to rigorous testing both for their efficacy and for their dangers. If, as has happened with some drugs, unacceptable side effects emerge in spite of this testing then the preparation is withdrawn. Psychiatrists should not use medications that have not met the standards of efficacy and safety laid down by law.

The basic principle of medicine is first to do no harm. It is often assumed that talking is always helpful and can never do harm. In recent years it has become apparent that talking therapies can indeed do harm. For example, there is convincing evidence that some of these treatments can provoke relapse in those with schizophrenia, especially when the talking therapy is of a very intense or analytic variety. There is also evidence that debriefing, the practice of reliving a traumatic experience so as to allow the ventilation of emotion, can also make psychiatric illness more likely following a major trauma.

One of the other problems about these therapies is that most have not been subject to the same tests for effectiveness as drug treatments. Those therapies that have include behaviour therapy, used for phobias, and cognitive therapy, used in mild to moderate depression. Family therapy is also helpful for those with schizophrenia who come from hostile families. It is possible that your nephew comes from a supportive family and that this is not necessary in his case.

Personnel Shortages

Most psychiatric units and out-patient departments now have clinical psychologists and behaviour therapists, as well as alcohol counsellors, working as part of the team to deliver a range of treatments. Unfortunately, in many parts of the country there is a shortage of these therapists. The issue is not that psychiatrists are uncomfortable working with those who practice psychotherapy in its various forms and indeed many psychiatrists have been trained in these techniques themselves. Ultimately, we must treat our patients with proven interventions as appropriate to the person's condition rather than with treatments that have popular appeal.

* * *

Schizophrenia is one of the illnesses that relapses unless appropriate medication is prescribed and there is no evidence to show that psychotherapy can replace medication in this condition, although in certain circumstances specific types of talking therapy may be combined with medication.

Useful Website

www.mentalhealth.com/dis/p20-ps01.html
(This is called the Internet Mental Health site)

Useful Contact

The Mental Health Association of Ireland
Tel. (01) 2841166

My son has schizophrenia and is being treated with tranquillizers, which he gets by injection every few weeks. I would much rather that he had counselling as I am worried that he will become addicted to his medication and that he will have trouble coming off it. Could I talk to his doctor about this?

The medications that are used in treating schizophrenia are called major tranquillizers. They are not addictive. In this respect, major tranquillizers differ from those termed minor tranquillizers that are used in everyday medical practice to treat anxiety, insomnia and tension. Since the medications your son is taking are not addictive he should have no trouble when the time comes to stop them.

Stopping Medication

It is unclear if it would be advisable for your son to stop his medication, as this depends on how many times he has been ill previously and on his symptoms. If this is his first episode of illness then he may be able to discontinue them in about two years – that is the recommended duration for the initial phase. If, however, he has experienced a relapse he may need them for much longer, perhaps indefinitely. A further consideration is the type of symptoms that he now has. If he is well with medication and able to go about his daily activities, such as work and so on, this is a good sign and again the possibility of stopping the medication at some point is realistic. However, if he is not coping with day-to-day activities well, if he is spending a lot of time in bed or if he appears to lack motivation, then coming off medication may not be advisable and a change of treatment may even be indicated to help these problems.

Positive and Negative Symptoms

Medication itself can sometimes cause lethargy and low mood. If so, a change would be helpful. However, it may not be the drugs that are causing apathy, low energy and disinterest but the illness itself. These features of schizophrenia are called the negative symptoms. These symptoms often persist after the others, known as positive symptoms (hearing voices and having unusual false beliefs), disappear. The newer medications used to treat this illness are particularly good at targeting both the negative and positive symptoms and should now be used as the first line treatment once the diagnosis is made.

Counselling

Unfortunately, on its own counselling has not been shown to be helpful in treating either the positive or negative symptoms of schizophrenia. That is not to say that your son should not receive help in dealing with his day-to-day problems but this should be in conjunction with medication. There is good research evidence that those with schizophrenia are at risk of relapsing if the therapy is very probing or intensive. The most appropriate approach is to be supportive and provide a listening ear. Educating your son about his illness would also be helpful.

Why Injections?

The injections which your son receives are known as depot injections and they are almost always given to those who are unreliable in taking their medication. By giving it in this form, a regular supply of treatment is ensured and relapse is prevented. It is of course best for the person's self-esteem to allow them to accept responsibility for taking medication, but ultimately this has to be measured against the risk of relapse. Injections may be more associated with side effects such as tremor, stiffness and restlessness, although by keeping the dose as low as possible these can be minimised. Also, following a change in dosage it takes longer to notice an effect, since treatment is given only every few weeks.

In spite of these problems there is good news for those who have to take their medication as an injection. There is now an injectable form of one of the newer medications available and this probably has fewer side effects. If your son is not happy with his medication at present he should discuss it with his psychiatrist and consider a change.

* * *

You can certainly speak to your son's psychiatrist about this but you will need your son's permission. Alternatively, you may wish to speak to his community nurse, since they probably give your son his injections. Again, you will need your son's permission. Schizophrenia Ireland offers excellent support to families and I strongly recommend that you contact them also.

Useful Reading

Mueser, K.T. and Gingrich, S. (1994) *Coping with Schizophrenia: A Guide for Families*, New Harbinger: Oakland, CA

Useful Contact

Schizophrenia Ireland
38 Blessington Street, Dublin 7, Tel. (01) 8601620, e-mail: schizi@iol.ie

I am twenty-one and have recently been diagnosed with schizophrenia. Thankfully, I am very well on medication and I have even returned to work. I am also going out with my friends again and they are very helpful and supportive, as are my parents. In spite of this I feel stigmatised, especially as I know how people regard schizophrenia. I am especially worried in case I will become violent or develop a "split personality". I also hate taking medication.

I am delighted that you are well again and back at work. Many people, perhaps even yourself when you were at the height of your illness, would not have believed that you could ever be well again. However, the newer medications that have become available in the last five or so years are excellent and, provided you continue to take them, you should remain well.

Is Medication Necessary?

It is tempting to discontinue treatment when you feel well and when you are back at routine activities again, such as work. This would be foolish, since you would relapse within a few months. Many people find taking medication a nuisance and wonder if some other approach, such as counselling, would be better. However, all the research to date shows that medication is essential to prevent relapse, for up to two years in the first instance. The first six months following recovery is the time when relapse is most likely. Research also shows that counselling may itself provoke recurrences by focussing intensely on thoughts and feelings.

Some people feel that they are less worthwhile as human beings if they require medication to stay well. However, most people with physical ailments such as high blood pressure or diabetes do not regard themselves as less valuable because they require medication in order to stay alive. Your illness is also a biological one and requires medication to treat it.

Unpredictable Behaviour

It must be very frightening, feeling that you might "snap" at any moment and lose control, as you suggest in your question. However, this is one of the myths associated with schizophrenia and with all psychiatric disorders. If your illness is controlled with medication then there is virtually no chance of this happening, provided you are not violent by nature. Such an occurrence is only possible if you are relapsing and even then it is unlikely.

Similarly, the view that "split personality" and schizophrenia are the same is also a myth. The split that occurs in schizophrenia is not of the personality but a separation from reality, so that the sufferer believes that they are being persecuted, that their thoughts are being controlled or that voices are speaking to them. These acute symptoms are very responsive to medication and fade usually after a few weeks.

Support from Others

It is great that you have the support of your friends and family. However, they must not be over-protective either. They can best help you by gently encouraging you to resume your former activities, but at your own pace. It would be harmful to you if they rushed you too much or if they were too watchful of you. In fact, families that are over-involved run the risk of provoking relapse. If you feel that your parents are excessively concerned about you, I suggest that you ask them to see your psychiatrist, if they have not already done so.

Overcoming Stigma

I accept that you feel stigmatised, but the best way to overcome this is by remaining well and by equipping yourself with accurate knowledge about your condition. It is probably too early yet, but in due course you might be in a position to speak to your close friends about the diagnosis and by so doing improve their knowledge of what schizophrenia is and is not.

* * *

By remaining well you will disprove some of the myths that stigmatise those with schizophrenia.

Useful Reading

The Schizophrenia Handbook (2002), published by Schizophrenia Ireland

Useful Website

www.schizophrenia.com

Useful Contact

Schizophrenia Ireland
38 Blessington Street, Dublin 7, Tel. (01) 8601620, e-mail: schizi@iol.ie

Somatoform Disorders

The mind has a great influence over the body and maladies often have their origin there.

Moliere,
Love's the Best Doctor, *trans. 1953*

Somatoform Disorders

I have often heard the term "malingering". I am not sure that I know exactly what it means but I think it implies that symptoms are made up. Is this correct? I have a colleague at work whom I think may be malingering following a minor car accident. She has all types of physical symptoms yet she also seems to enjoy going out and is able to come to work as usual. I am angry to think that she may be magnifying her difficulties for financial reasons and I am tempted to challenge her about it.

Your description of malingering is correct. Essentially, it is characterised by the production of false or grossly exaggerated symptoms, physical or psychological, for some form of personal gain. This may be financial such as compensation, or it may be to avoid some difficult or dangerous situation, such as army postings. Sometimes people malinger as a way of retaliating against another when the person feels wronged. It is impossible to provide a figure for its prevalence but doctors and lawyers know that it is common.

Seeking Compensation

The most common situation in which malingering takes place is when there is a legal claim and compensation is being considered for personal injury. Following car accidents or other personal injuries, for instance, symptoms may be produced or exaggerated. It is found most commonly in settings with a preponderance of men. For example, among army personnel, symptoms may be produced to avoid being posted away from home or to war-torn areas. Among prisoners, additional comforts may be provided on production of symptoms – moving to the sick bay and out of the cell. Sometimes those being sent for trial try to avoid this by feigning "madness".

Vague Symptoms

The symptoms may be physical or psychiatric and are generally vague and difficult to refute. For example, headache, dizziness, pain in the back, chest or abdomen, depression and forgetfulness are commonly described. Usually the person will tell you that they find the symptoms unpleasant, uncomfortable and distressing. However, on all objective testing this does not seem correct, since the malingerer usually goes about other aspects of life normally, such as going out socially, taking an interest in day-to-day matters and so on.

Fooling Doctors

It seems incredible but doctors can sometimes be fooled into accepting the patients' symptoms without question. However, the underlying principle of the doctor-patient relationship is that it is based on trust – a trust that the patient is genuinely suffering and that the doctor will do their best to alleviate this suffering. Malingering is totally at odds with this principle and doctors are therefore reluctant to believe that a patient may be less than honest about symptoms.

As the doctor gets to know the patient it may become increasingly clear that the symptoms are deliberately being made up or exaggerated for external gain. Unfortunately, the problem of malingering is likely to increase now that so many people have access to the Internet and can download the symptoms of a variety of conditions.

Confrontation

It is understandable that you are tempted to confront your colleague at work but I would strongly suggest you do not. Firstly, you do not know that she is definitely malingering. She may have genuine difficulties and may be struggling to cope with life, putting on a brave face at work and with her friends. It is well recognised that physical symptoms can be of psychological origin, especially following accidents. If you confront her, your relationship with her will certainly deteriorate and this will make working with her difficult. I suggest you avoid talking about her symptoms at all and instead focus on other things.

* * *

It is unfortunate that some people are not as honest as we would wish them to be, but then humanity is imperfect.

Useful Website
www.psychological.com/malingering.htm

Somatoform Disorders

For years my sister has been complaining of physical ailments. She is frequently admitted to hospital and has even had operations to treat her symptoms. I believe she is making these up but she manages to deceive the doctors. She has only just been referred to a psychiatrist who says she has Munchausen's syndrome. Can you tell me about this condition?

The history that you tell me is typical of Munchausen's syndrome. The disorder is named after the German Baron von Munchausen, who lived in the 18th century and wrote many travel and adventure stories. Other names for the condition are hospital addiction and professional patient syndrome.

Feigning Symptoms

Like your sister, patients with this condition have numerous admissions to hospital with various physical symptoms. They can feign symptoms of many diseases and will be very familiar with a variety of disorders. Indeed, so convincing is their history that even very experienced clinicians can be deceived, as they seem to have been in regard to your sister. One of the problems is that when the patient presents to casualty some of the physical investigations may be abnormal, as urine is often deliberately contaminated or bleeding may have been self-induced. Sometimes the patient may use drugs such as insulin to induce coma. Many patients have multiple scars on their abdomen from the myriad of surgical procedures that they have undergone.

Demanding

Not surprisingly, these patients are very demanding when they are in hospital and once admitted frequently demand specific drugs. Many are dependent on prescribed drugs. It is commonly the case that they threaten litigation when, in their eyes, their symptoms are not being correctly diagnosed or treated. Most problematic of all is that they often discharge themselves from hospital when the medical team is on the point of deciding that their symptoms are false. They then go to another hospital and the cycle begins again.

Sick Role

The core of the disorder is that the symptoms are knowingly fabricated for the purpose of being looked after – in other words it is the sick role and the attention attached to it that drives the behaviour. For this reason it is crucial that the behaviour is not encouraged or reinforced by actually admitting the person to hospital. Many such patients have a history of lengthy periods of childhood illness and wish to return to that period in their lives when they were looked after and cosseted. So although the symptoms are deliberately exaggerated, the motivation comes from an inner need to be cared for rather than the external desire for financial gain, as happens in malingering.

Munchausen's by Proxy

This is a condition in which a person, usually a mother, either fabricates symptoms in her child or induces symptoms such as vomiting, rashes and so on for the purpose of seeing her child investigated and receive treatment. This provides her with a sense of purpose and as with Munchausen's syndrome, the proxy variety is also motivated by her needs rather than that of the child. It was first described in 1977 by a paediatrician in Britain and it has recently received considerable media attention.

It is a controversial diagnosis that many question. One of the problems is that there is little scientific literature on this topic and the diagnosis seems to be made on the basis of excluding physical causes for the child's problem rather than on any positive features. Indeed, some of the features of this condition are contradictory – the observation that the parent is angry about the child's condition or not upset enough. When this "diagnosis" is made the child is invariably removed from the mother.

Help

Unfortunately, there is no specific treatment for Munchausen's syndrome and the focus is on containment. General support as well as treatment of any associated drug addictions are necessary, although establishing a good therapeutic relationship with these patients is very difficult, as they see the role of psychiatrists being primarily to prevent them getting the attention they so badly crave.

It is crucial also that general medical staff does not show anger and resentment towards those patients with Munchausen's syndrome or with Munchausen's by Proxy, although these emotions are understandable. Also, confronting and humiliating the patient can lead to abrupt discharge, only for the behaviour to be repeated in another hospital. Unfortunately, there is very little research available on the best treatments, although clearly confrontation is not advisable.

* * *

I cannot give you much optimism about your sister's condition. I hope you can persuade her to continue to see the psychiatrist who may at least be able to reframe her need as a "cry for help" rather than as a malicious attempt to deceive her doctors. You too should take this line with her, although it may be very draining for you and you may feel enraged with her at times.

Useful Website

www.priory.com/psych/factitious.htm

Stress

All stress is bad.

Common myth

I have been hearing and reading a lot about stress recently and I really don't know what it means. Surely everybody is stressed at some time. I have a very challenging job and a family also and people often ask me if I'm stressed. I can honestly say that I feel overloaded at times but I am also very happy and fulfilled. Am I suffering with stress?

Stress is an all-encompassing word that, as you say, is talked about rather a lot these days. The definition of stress is that it is the process that occurs as individuals adapt to or deal with circumstances that threaten to disrupt their physical or psychological functioning. This means that the body and mind are provided with a reminder that their well-being is under threat from some event or situation. The latter is termed the stressor. Common stressors are those that involve change, loss, frustration, boredom, pressure, fear or trauma and the more stressors that occur in a short space of time the more likely is the person to suffer physical or psychological symptoms. Most people recognise that time pressures and over-work can cause problems but few recognise that boredom from lack of stimulation can be an equally damaging stressor. Burn-out, the loss of function and exhaustion that results from a continuous flow of stressors are forms of stress reaction that many in demanding jobs, as you describe yours to be, experience.

Normal versus Abnormal Stress

Unfortunately, the term stress has such negative connotations that it is thought to warrant some type of help, even when the reactions are understandable and normal. So any unpleasant emotion such as feeling upset after a loss or feeling apprehensive about a new job are regarded by some as evidence of an abnormality and of the need for treatment to remove these feelings. This is an incorrect understanding of stress.

The distinction between normal stress and that which is abnormal is crucial, however, since no intervention is required for normal reactions whereas abnormal stress should not be allowed to continue indefinitely. In some situations a degree of stress is beneficial, "psyching up" to the task that is to be performed – for example the surgeon performing an operation might become slip-shod if they didn't feel some apprehension or the student preparing for an examination might be less inclined to study if they did not worry about the result.

The distinction between normal and abnormal stress is dependent on the extent to which these symptoms effect functioning and health. When the stress level is so high that day-to-day functioning is impaired or that physical and/or psychological health is adversely affected then the stress reaction is regarded as abnormal. If your functioning is adversely affected by the pressures you are experiencing at home and at work then your are suffering from abnormal stress and need professional help.

Manifestations

The features of stress, whether normal or abnormal, are most often psychological, such as feeling sad, tense, fearful, worried etc. However, it is only when functioning such as the ability to get to work, or do it properly is impaired that professional help is required.

Sometimes abnormal stress may tip over into depressive illness or anxiety disorders. Physical symptoms can occur also and these include loss of appetite, poor sleep, aches and pains and breathing difficulties. Blood pressure may also rise and ulcers can develop. Overwhelming stress can lead to post-traumatic stress disorder. Finally, stress may show itself in day-to-day behaviour with irritability, absenteeism from work, increased alcohol consumption, poor time keeping and at times overdosing or even suicide.

Why Do People React Differently?

There is also a personal element to the development of abnormal stress: if two people are exposed to an identical stressor, both may react differently, one coping well and the other having serious problems with functioning. The factors that influence the individual reaction to an event are known as mediators and include personality, coping skills, chemical vulnerability to anxiety or depression, religious beliefs and the support system that is in place.

Among the positive coping skills are confronting rather than avoiding the problem. So taking a holiday when a significant stressor is present is not likely to be helpful – better defer the holiday until the problem has resolved. Having friends to talk to, as you have, is also helpful but research shows that their support is best used, not as a shoulder to cry on, although this can be helpful in the short term, but for practical assistance and advice in resolving the difficulty. Some people find prayer very helpful and meditation such as yoga is helpful in bringing about relaxation. Among the negative coping skills are drinking alcohol to reduce the symptoms, putting the problem on the long finger and distracting oneself from the difficulty by constant activity.

* * *

The distinction between normal and abnormal stress is crucial and one that is often overlooked. In your case, I suggest you visit your general practitioner to have your situation assessed.

> **Useful Website**
>
> www.ivf.com/stress.html

I have been reading a lot about depression recently and I am very confused about the causes. I read that stresses such as changing jobs or moving house could trigger it, yet everybody suffers stress at some time in their life but not everyone needs treatment for depression. For example, my mother died last year and I was very upset, yet I never regarded myself as suffering with depression or needing treatment. Can you clarify what the situation is please?

You are correct – it is confusing and most people who have stressful events in their life do not suffer with depression as a result, nor do they need any special help in coping other than general support and advice from family and friends. However, life stresses can affect some people badly by causing severe or prolonged symptoms for which help may be needed.

Depressive Illness

There is a large volume of research into the role of life events in triggering depressive illness and it confirms that the six months following the event is the time of greatest risk. In particular events such as moving house, changing job, being bereaved, experiencing loss of any type and a host of others may actually be the stimulus for a depressive illness. Pleasant events can also lead to depressive illness, in particular childbirth.

Especially vulnerable to the negative effect of these events are those who are isolated and who do not have support from family. Personality is also important and people who find change difficult may develop depression in the face of an event associated with change. Also, those who are very dependent on others may become clinically depressed when that support is removed. For example, a parent who is very dependent on a child or a spouse who relies excessively on their partner may become depressed if the child moves away from home or the partner dies.

Unhappiness

It is also recognised that many, probably most people are unhappy for periods in their lives when problems arise. As you point out, there is usually no need for professional help. Mostly, when people are unhappy they continue to function normally; others have problems functioning but do eventually adjust to the stressful situation. These are said to be suffering stress reactions. However, there are some who do not adjust and who have trouble even doing the routine chores – this is the group that has clinical depression. The problem is that distinguishing clinical depression, termed depressive illness, from stress reactions can be difficult, as the symptoms are similar and there is no chemical test that can be used to assist. However, waking early in the morning and being unable to return to sleep, as well as feeling worse in the morning are uncommon in those who are unhappy and stressed as distinct from those who have a clinical depression.

Vulnerability

It is clear then that events can provoke depressive illness, stress reactions or short-term understandable reactions that resolve spontaneously. Many assume that having counselling in regard to such an event will prevent these reactions recurring. Unfortunately, this is not the case: whilst it may be helpful in the short term to explore the issue in therapy, this does not prevent recurrences. So, when a depressive illness arises following, for example, a job loss, episodes of depression may later arise without any provocation. This seems to defy logic but there is a large body of research involving following up those with depression that demonstrates this. Biological sensitisation is the phrase that is used to describe this phenomenon.

Complex Interaction

It is clear that the manner in which stressful events trigger stress reactions and depression is complex and involves an interaction between the events, the personality of the individual and the background support and relationships that are available. A final piece in this jigsaw is genetic-predisposition and there are some who have an innate vulnerability to depressive illness that manifests itself when the combination of stressful events, personality, support systems and individual predisposition is present. For these reasons, some people can deal with major traumatic events except for a period of unhappiness that passes; others show signs of stress; and still others become ill and need treatment.

* * *

You are fortunate that you belong to the first group and ride the problems that life brings you without any more serious consequences.

Useful Reading

Bates, Tony (1999) *Depression: The Common Sense Approach*, New Leaf: Dublin

Salmans, Sandra (1997) *Depression: Questions you Have, Answers you Need*, Thorsons: London

---

I recently got the promotion at work that I had dreamed of but it isn't working out as well as I expected. Also, my brother is very ill in hospital and my fiancée and I have just split up. I feel so alone as my brother and I were very close and I can't tell him about my problems when he is sick. I have been crying a lot and not able to sleep. My doctor, who is wonderful, suggested that I take antidepressants. I am reluctant because I know I will feel better when these problems have gone.

You certainly have more than your fill of worries and it is hardly surprising that you have trouble adjusting to your new role at work. It is also to be expected that with so many worries you will be tearful and upset. In particular, the understandable absence of your brother's support is creating a vacuum in your life that makes it difficult for you to cope at present, not to mention your worries about his illness. However, as these difficulties resolve, your mood should improve in parallel.

Regrettably, many doctors nowadays seem to think that antidepressants are the solution to all of life's problems – they are not. Antidepressants are excellent at treating clinical depression and, used properly, they can renew life for the depressed person but they are not useful in eliminating our understandable reactions to day-to-day problems.

Clinical Depression

Your symptoms seem appropriate to your circumstances and what you feel is not abnormal at all, since this seems to have arisen at an upsetting and challenging time in your life. In fact, you have had three major stressors in recent weeks. Even if you took an antidepressant it probably would not do any good and you might experience side effects such as feeling slightly spaced out, dizzy or nauseated.

Unfortunately, a small proportion of those who experience these types of negative events go on to develop clinical depression. In other words, they move from unhappiness to illness and the mood change persists even when pleasant things happen. The result is that any attempt to improve the feelings of sadness, such as having a holiday, make no difference nor does the depressed feeling improve when the stressful situation is resolved. If you had a clinical depression, the return of your fiancée or an improvement in your brother's health would make no difference to your emotions. In such circumstances antidepressants are very helpful.

The typical symptoms of clinical depression include waking early in the morning, feeling worse first thing in the morning, loss of interest in usual activities and feelings of guilt and hopelessness. Your doctor will be the best person to make an assessment in the first instance as to whether you have a clinical depression or a stress disorder.

Symptom Relief

Some symptoms of stress, as distinct from clinical depression, may benefit from chemical treatments in the short term. Sleeping tablets may help, but first you should try "sleep hygiene" measures such as avoiding caffeine or nicotine at night, taking a milky drink before bed and limiting exercise to early in the evening rather than before bedtime. Relaxation exercises before settling for the night are helpful. If these approaches do not work then a sleeping tablet, for short-term use, might improve sleep, since lack of sleep worsens feelings of despondency and gloom and increases irritability. If you do take sleeping tablets they should not be prescribed on a regular basis for more than four weeks. Also, do not be tempted to drink to relieve your distress – unfortunately, many people do so at difficult times such as you are experiencing at present.

Self-Help

It is important to make space for yourself at present and try to limit the demands upon your time, as far as possible. Some people get great comfort from reading spiritual or self-help books, from prayer, meditation or from just sitting and being still. Ultimately, in coping with your present problems you must draw on your inner reserves of insight, instinct and common sense. You will also have to rely on the support of others more than you are perhaps used to and it might help you to see a professional counsellor if you are unable to confide in your family or friends.

* * *

If you are in doubt about taking an antidepressant, and from your story I believe that your doubts are well founded, then you should ask for a second opinion. I hope that your problems resolve soon and that life can get back on an even keel.

Useful Reading

Weekes, Claire (1995) *Self-Help for your Nerves*, Harper Collins: London

Useful Website

www.nlm.nih.gov/medlineplus/anxiety.html

I am forty-six and work in an office where I hold a very senior position. I feel that I am suffering from stress as I am overloaded with work, I have several meetings every day and I can barely catch up with paper work. Sometimes I don't even have time for a coffee break or lunch and I frequently have to bring work home. I have started taking time off work due to exhaustion. I am having trouble sleeping and I worry all the time. Can I do anything about it?

It seems that you may be suffering from abnormal stress, since your performance and behaviour are now being affected by your work overload. Many people describe similar symptoms to you yet do not recognise the cause – the fact that you have identified the problem is a very positive first step. There are several approaches to dealing with your problem.

Attacking the Stressor

Abnormal stress is caused by events and situations that are termed stressors. Avoiding these, if possible, is important. In your case your workload is the main factor, since you seem to have little time for anything else. So saying "no" to requests to take on even more work is something that we find difficult but is important. You should also consider if extra help is needed due to staff shortages and, if so, rectify this. If you cannot decline extra work you should ask yourself why – is it because you are hard on yourself, because you feel nobody can do it as well as you or because you have nobody to delegate it to? If you are asking colleagues or other assistants to help, you must be able to trust that person to do the work competently. If you cannot, then your level of tension and worry will increase further and you would need to discuss the situation with management.

When people are stressed they tend to feel overwhelmed, unable to see the wood for the trees, and they try to solve everything at once. You should prioritise the problems you are experiencing in terms of the ease with which they can be resolved and their importance. Are meetings a bigger problem than paper work? If so, focus on these – one at a time.

A piecemeal, structured approach such as this is useful. It is helpful to make a "To do" list each morning and give your attention to each item on the list in order of urgency and importance. A timetable for each day will also help you focus on particular tasks at specific times, so you will not be worrying that some are untouched and decisions not made, as each will have its allocated time.

If you do not take breaks for lunch and tea then your efficiency, not to mention your blood sugar, will drop and so too will your output. Therefore, you must ensure that you take these breaks to allow yourself to recharge physically and psychologically. It might also be a good idea to monitor your efficiency, since you may be spending too much time talking or making telephone calls instead of focusing on the job in hand.

Focusing on Mediators

Not everybody who has problems at work or at home develops abnormal stress. This is because of factors that influence our reactions and these include having support from those close to us. In your case there may be colleagues who can help or your spouse may also be glad to assist, particularly if your family has felt excluded recently. Initially, you will find it useful to talk and offload your worries, but the effects of this are likely to be short lived. Ultimately, the benefits of support from others come from the assistance they give in finding solutions to the difficulties. Speak only to a few trusted mentors, otherwise you may get conflicting advice and become even more uncertain about solutions. As these present themselves, it is important to systematically weigh up the advantages and disadvantages of each, if necessary by outlining the options and their feasibility in writing.

Symptom Reduction

The symptoms caused by the stressors can be targeted. In your case, the main effects are tension, exhaustion and worry. Periods of relaxation and quietness are important if you want to avoid burn-out. So having coffee breaks, limiting the amount of time you spend on work at home and so on become vital. Exercise, listening to music or taking a relaxing bath with salts and candles will also help you unwind. Alcohol in moderation can be a relaxant, but be careful that you control the amount you drink. Yoga is beneficial for many and some people get great comfort from praying. Tranquillizers may be useful in the short term but they should not be taken indefinitely. It is best to try to resolve the cause of your abnormal stress. You may find that having dealt with one aspect of the stressor such as the excess of meetings you will not be so overwhelmed by the others and that you will have more mental energy to devote to their resolution.

Finally, having time for yourself each day will allow you the personal space to evaluate how you are dealing with your difficulties and to generate alternative strategies. This will also remove you from the treadmill of work and worry.

* * *

If these simple techniques do not work and you are still excessively tense you should consult your doctor.

Useful Website

www.teachhealth.com

Substance Abuse

There is increasing recognition of the impact of substance misuse on individuals and society ... Services should be able to respond to a spectrum of need and should work closely with, and in support of, primary care, other secondary care services, and non-statutory agencies.

Royal College of Psychiatrists, London
Council Report, 2002

My son is twenty-five and has a good job. He lives at home but recently I have noticed that he goes to the pub most nights. He never did that before, as he loved to play sport in the evenings. He also goes to the off-licence and brings home cans. I've noticed that he is having trouble getting up in the mornings and I know that his boss has reprimanded him for his poor time keeping. He seems to have lost interest in sport and he is argumentative with the others in the family. I worry that he may be an alcoholic. What can I do?

It seems that your son does have serious problems with alcohol as it is taking over his life. He is beginning to forego his hobbies in favour of alcohol and it appears to be playing an increasingly important role in his life. It is common for those who drink too much to have trouble getting up in the morning and so poor time keeping and even absenteeism become problems. Your son is running the risk of losing his job if this continues.

Undesirable Effects

The fact that he is argumentative may be one of the recognised undesirable effects of alcohol. Alcohol removes the inhibitions that we normally have and instead of "holding our tongue" when we are irritated we show our annoyance. His argumentativeness may also be an indication of his annoyance with his own behaviour, which he is directing at you. Have you noticed any other symptoms in your son, such as gloominess or incontinence of urine? Unfortunately, bladder control is poor in those who abuse alcohol and because it is embarrassing, it is not admitted. Many who abuse alcohol complain that they feel very gloomy and hopeless and in a small proportion this may require specific treatment. For over 90 per cent, the low mood is due to the direct effect of alcohol on the brain and it lifts when drinking ceases.

Dependence

As alcohol abuse becomes established, the person has to increase the amount of alcohol they drink in order to obtain the same effect, i.e. their tolerance increases. This leads to the consumption of large quantities of alcohol, eventually affecting the liver. In the early stages of alcohol dependence it may be possible to just stop drinking without any difficulty. However, once the person has become physically, as distinct from psychologically, dependent then some unpleasant and dangerous symptoms occur and the detoxification must take place in hospital. This takes about one week.

Needing Help

Have you or any of your family discussed your concern with him? He may disagree and say he is drinking no more than others in his circle of friends. This is an excuse that is often used to justify the high consumption but you could point out that unlike his friends he now appears to be having work-related problems. If he will not listen to you then a family member or friend whom he trusts might speak with him. He should be encouraged to go to his family doctor, or to AA (Alcoholics Anonymous) although he may find this too threatening right now. There are also many residential centres available for the treatment of those with alcohol problems. I am sometimes asked if compulsory admission for treatment is possible but this is not regarded as a good idea, since ultimately the success of treatment depends on your son's motivation.

Treatment Options

You may be tempted to try to find out why he is drinking so much, but I feel this would be unhelpful, since the priority is to persuade him that he has a problem and that he needs to stop. During the treatment period with the counsellor after detoxification, the cause of his alcohol abuse, if any, as well as lifestyle changes that he needs to make will be explored. He may also be prescribed a drug called disulfiram. This is a prop for those who are impulsively tempted to resume drinking, since it causes nausea and vomiting when taken with alcohol. There is also a new drug, called acamprosate, available to help reduce craving, although none of these are effective on their own, unless combined with alcohol counselling.

There are also options that you might find personally helpful. Al-anon offers support for family members, which is particularly important for you at present when you probably feel desperate about your son's situation.

* * *

Finally, it may not be helpful to use the term "alcoholic", as this word conjures up images of people on skid row having lost everything. It is better to talk about alcohol problems rather than risk alienating him at this point.

Useful Reading

Steinglass, P., Bennett, L.A., Wolin, S.J. and Reiss, D. (1993) *The Alcoholic Family*, Basic Books: New York

Useful Website

www.alcoholmd.com

Useful Contacts

Alcoholics Anonymous
109 South Circular Road, Dublin 8, Tel. (01) 4538998

Al-Anon
5 Capel Street, Dublin 1, Tel. (01) 8732699

My son is an alcoholic but he is doing nothing about looking for help. I often wonder if he is also taking drugs. He lies in bed all day and stays out all hours of the night. He has a university degree but doesn't use it and is now on the dole. He was engaged to be married last year to a lovely girl but she couldn't put up with his apathy and his refusal to do anything about his problems so she broke off the relationship. My husband and I have discussed the possibility of certifying him to a psychiatric unit but we don't know how to go about it. Can you help?

You must feel very frustrated that your son is wasting his ability, his life and his money on alcohol and possibly drugs. I can understand why you feel certification and compulsory treatment may be the answer. However, I do not think that forcing your son into treatment is the correct approach.

Danger

In general, a person is forced to have treatment only if they are a danger to self or others. This means that the behaviour of the person poses an immediate threat to life, either their own through suicide or others' through violence stemming from the underlying psychiatric disorder. Also, if the psychiatric condition of a patient is at risk of deteriorating this might constitute grounds for compulsory admission. Your son's ongoing problem with alcohol does not come within these parameters, although there are some circumstances in which certification might be justified.

Process

If your son became suicidal and was refusing treatment you might have grounds for certification. This is a three-stage process. The first stage would involve you or some family member making an application for his compulsory detention. Then a doctor, usually the person's general practitioner but sometimes a casualty officer if the person is seen in the accident department, signs the medical recommendation. This must be done within twenty-four hours of examining the patient. At this point a second opinion from a different general practitioner must be offered to the patient and whilst some patients eagerly accept this, others do not want it. Finally, the psychiatrist makes the decision and completes the third part of the form, accepting the patient if there is a clinical indication for this. Sometimes the psychiatrist declines to complete this if their opinion is that compulsory admission in the circumstances is not required or if the patient agrees to come to hospital voluntarily.

Legal Protection

If the patient feels that the detention is illegal then an application can be made for judicial review through the hospital administration or through a solicitor. Under new legislation it is proposed that there will be an automatic review of the legality of the procedure within twenty-eight days of admission. At present, most compulsory admissions last less than fourteen days because with improvement in the psychiatric condition the person is no longer a threat to self or to others.

Careful Consideration

You will appreciate that the method of bringing about a compulsory admission is not straightforward and is governed by law with respect to the rights of the person being certified. I suspect that you would find it difficult to find a psychiatrist willing to accept your son, at present, as a compulsory patient. The other difficulty with such admissions is that following treatment and discharge there is often huge resentment and anger on the part of the detained person towards the family member initiating the admission. In your son's case, where his recovery depends specifically on his own motivation rather than on taking medication, this is likely to be a particularly difficult problem. I would urge you to first discuss your proposal with your family doctor.

* * *

Ultimately, it is your son who will have to make the decision to deal with his alcohol abuse. There are no easy answers and certification is probably not the solution.

Useful Contact
Irish Council for Civil Liberties
Tel. (01) 6779813

My husband is a very heavy drinker. He often misses work, especially on a Monday morning, and I have to telephone and make excuses for him. I sometimes go out to the pub with him, just to keep an eye on him and to drive home, but I have given up saying anything about his drinking as he just gets annoyed with me. What can I do?

I am sorry you have this problem. It can be very difficult making somebody accept that alcohol may be a problem. However, the fact that he misses work because of drinking is an indicator of the seriousness of his difficulty.

Collusion

I know it is tempting to go out with him to check on how much he drinks, but in doing this you are to some extent colluding with his behaviour. Do you ever buy alcohol for him? This is something that family members also do and again this is unintentionally re-enforcing the behaviour. Of course, he might have an accident and I can understand why you would want to do everything that you can to prevent this. However, your husband is an adult and you cannot be responsible for him.

One of the things you should do is stop making excuses for his absences from work. Again, in doing this you are allowing him "get away with" this unacceptable behaviour. You must tell him that from now on you will not go out with him nor will you facilitate him with any excuses that he makes to others about his drink.

Children

You do not say if you have children or what age they are. If they are young then they may be adversely affected by your husband's drink problem. Seeing their father in bed on Monday mornings is a very bad example for them. Moreover, if they witness regular rows between you and your husband they may come to resent him and if he is ever violent to you in front of them this may set the tone for how they relate to others later in life. So, for their sake, it is important to deal with his problem.

Resentment

The alcoholic is often the last person to accept the problem, especially when it is a spouse or close family member that suggests it, and this can cause huge resentment. Is there someone he particularly respects – what about your children (if they are adult) or his family? If so, then perhaps you could ask them to support you in your efforts to persuade him to get help. Maybe he has a friend from work whose help you could also look for in this delicate matter. Alternatively, his general practitioner might be told, so that he can raise it with your husband when he next visits – you could suggest to your husband that he goes for a general medical check-up.

Secrecy

The burden of alcohol abuse is often shouldered alone and kept a secret from everybody. However, if your husband will not take your advice, then you have no choice but to confide in others about it – that, or just put up with the unsatisfactory situation that presently prevails. I know you may feel it is a matter between both of you and you may even feel disloyal in discussing it with others but, ultimately, if his absenteeism continues he may loose his job. He will also damage his health.

The term alcoholic is one that is often shunned by those with drink problems, as it conjures up very disturbing images. However, it is a convenient shorthand term for alcohol dependence. If you or your husband do not want to use it then that's fine – provided help is sought.

* * *

At this point it is crucial that you resist the urge to take responsibility for him and that you enlist help in persuading him to give up and share your burden with others.

Useful Reading

Steinglass, P., Bennett, L.A., Wolin, S.J. and Reiss, D. (1993) *The Alcoholic Family*, Basic Books: New York

Useful Website

www.AlcoholMD.com

Useful Contacts

Alcoholics Anonymous
109 South Circular Road, Dublin 8, Tel. (01) 4538998

Al-Anon
5 Capel Street, Dublin 1, Tel. (01) 8732699

I know that I have a problem with alcohol because I drink as much as my money allows me every day. This is about seven pints. My doctor has suggested that I go into hospital to dry out, as I have been unable to do it myself. I am scared that this will be difficult for me and especially that I won't be able to remain abstinent afterwards. What help is available to me?

It is very good that you are thinking in this positive way, since motivation is the key to seeking treatment and remaining abstinent. Seven pints every day is indeed excessive – this is ninety-eight units per week (one unit is half a pint) and the maximum safe intake is twenty-one units per week.

Drying Out

If you go into hospital for drying out (detoxification) you will be put on medication to prevent serious withdrawal symptoms such as fits and confusion. Without this medication you would be at risk of developing delirium tremens (the DTs), a condition that must be avoided, as it can lead to death in up to 15 per cent of people. However, with medication, this condition will not occur and even though people feel generally unwell and may crave alcohol during the period of detoxification, most are able to cope with this discomfort. The detoxification process takes about ten to fourteen days and as the days pass, the medication will be reduced and you should be off it by the time you are discharged. You will also be given vitamin supplements, since the B group are often deficient in those who drink to excess.

Depression

Depressed mood is a frequent problem for those who drink to excess or abuse alcohol and this may be to the fore during withdrawal, since the short-term prop that alcohol provided is removed. However, alcohol is also a depressant so your mood should improve during the period of withdrawal, although you may not have returned fully to your old self by the time of discharge – this can take up to one month. Antidepressants are not usually required when low mood is associated with alcohol.

During your short hospitalisation you will receive one-to-one counselling from the nurses or from the alcohol counsellor.

Staying Dry

Unfortunately, the detoxification period is the easiest part of controlling alcoholism and following discharge, once the support and encouragement that is experienced in hospital is removed, many relapse and begin drinking again. To prevent this, continuing counselling is imperative, since it will educate you about alcohol; more importantly it will help you to identify triggers to your drinking behaviour. You will be helped to find other strategies for dealing with stresses in your life if these are thought to be important contributors to your excessive drinking.

Some people benefit from "antabuse", also called disulfiram. By causing nausea and vomiting when taken with alcohol it acts as a deterrent in those who drink impulsively. So it can be helpful in preventing sudden binges. Of course, if you decide to stop taking it you would be able to drink without any unpleasant effects – its use is in supporting motivation. There is also a drug available that reduces craving and this is helpful in many people. However, both of these drugs are only effective in the long term if combined with counselling. You may find AA helpful – some derive great benefit from this organisation, while others are uncomfortable disclosing their personal stories. I suggest you attend a few meetings, as you will undoubtedly get huge support and you will see that it is possible to become dry and stay that way.

Always an Alcoholic

Many think that at a special time there is no harm in one drink. However, the maxim "once an alcoholic, always an alcoholic" is worth bearing in mind and one that you have probably heard before and will hear many times again. Although about 10 per cent of problem drinkers do return to controlled drinking, you are almost certainly not in that group as your problem is very severe. You must get used to being alcohol-free for an indefinite period.

Complications

Many people do not realise that alcohol, taken to excess, can lead to serious complications. You probably know about liver disease, but it can also cause dementia due to the toxic effect on brain cells and there is a high risk of suicide also. Approximately 15 per cent of alcoholics die in this way. You may not be aware of the negative effect alcoholism has on families, especially on children. These will be explored with you in therapy.

* * *

It is wonderful that you are seeking treatment and I wish you well.

Useful Reading

Alcohol our Favourite Drug, Royal College of Psychiatrists, Public Education Department: London

Useful Website

www.rcpsych.ac.uk
(Click on Mental Health Information)

Useful Contacts

Alcoholics Anonymous
109 South Circular Road, Dublin 8, Tel. (01) 4538998

Alcoholism Treatment Centre
Stanhope Street, Dublin 7, Tel. (01) 6673965

My boyfriend is twenty-three and he smokes a lot of cannabis with his friends. I refuse to take any as I am totally against drugs. Over the past six months or so he smokes every day and he says it's a harmless pastime, safer than drinking and that everybody is doing it. He is now out of work and doesn't seem interested in looking for any either. Is he right? Is cannabis harmless?

Your boyfriend is incorrect when he tells you that cannabis is harmless, although there is a grain of truth when he says that it is commonly used. In the United States it is the most widely used illicit substance. In the eighteen to twenty-five age group: over 50 per cent have used it at least once and about 20 per cent are current users. Even among younger teenagers, between twelve and seventeen, up to 15 per cent have used it once. These figures, high though they are, represent a decline from its peak use in the 1970s.

Cancer Risk

Cannabis is associated with a number of worrying problems and you are right to refuse to take it. The most serious potential adverse effect comes from the inhalation of cancer-inducing chemicals, similar to those in conventional tobacco. Heavy users are at risk of chronic chest disease and of lung cancer. Some studies also suggest that regular use of cannabis causes brain cells to die and reduces the level of the male hormone testosterone, leading to sterility, although more research is needed to confirm these findings.

Depression and Panic

The euphoria that cannabis induces is the principal reason for its use. Skills such as driving cars and operating machinery are impaired for up to twelve hours afterwards and so it resembles alcohol in this regard, making driving dangerous. If cannabis is combined with alcohol the effects are even worse due to the combined effects of each on the brain.

Another problem associated with use of cannabis is that once the feelings of contentment and happiness have worn off, the mood changes to one of depression and gloom, especially in heavy users. Some people describe paranoid thoughts and the belief that others are trying to harm them. These may be very prominent and prolonged in some users and may culminate in a condition known as cannabis psychosis for which a period of treatment in hospital may be required. Feelings of panic are also common in those using cannabis, even in moderation.

Other effects are lack of drive and difficulty in sustaining tasks either at school or work. This is known as an amotivational syndrome and may explain your boyfriend's reluctance to look for work. Your boyfriend also runs the risk of getting flashbacks, especially if he uses other illicit drugs.

Psychological Dependence

One of the dangers of regular cannabis use is that tolerance to the effects occurs, so that it is necessary to increase the amount smoked in order to achieve the same effect. If your boyfriend wishes to achieve a state of relaxation he will have to smoke more. Ultimately, he will find it difficult to refrain from his habit. Heavy use can cause cannabis intoxication with a heightened awareness of colour, sound and detail. Time also appears slow and there may be feelings of detachment and out-of-body experiences.

The psychological dependence that cannabis users experience is the most difficult aspect of giving up; there is no definite evidence of any physical withdrawal. In this respect, cannabis differs from opiate drugs such as heroin, which is associated with severe physical symptoms on withdrawal. This does not mean that giving up is easy – it is not, but it can be done with support and determination.

* * *

You are quite right to be concerned about your boyfriend's use of cannabis. It is not harmless and he is fooling himself if he thinks it is.

Useful Websites

www.cannabis.net

www.eurad.net

Useful Contact

Drug Treatment Centre
30/31 Pearse Street, Dublin 2, Tel. (01) 6771122

I am twenty-five and single. I go to a lot of parties at weekends and there is a lot of cocaine circulating at them. Many of my friends take it and tell me the effect is wonderful. I would love to try it but I've never taken drugs before and I'm a little apprehensive. Is cocaine safe? My friends assure me that it is and that it's fine for recreational use.

Your friends are wrong and you are right to be very cautious. Cocaine is one of the most addictive and dangerous drugs and you should give it a wide berth. It is most commonly taken by snorting in powder form and amphetamines are often mixed in with the powder. Occasionally, it is injected intravenously. Crack-cocaine, a form of cocaine, is also very dangerous.

Glamour Drug

For many, cocaine has an air of glamour about it, as it seems to have for your friends. It was touted as a cure for many ills following its identification in 1860. Freud, the founder of psychoanalysis, snorted cocaine regularly. Scott Fitzgerald, the writer, wrote it into some of his novels. However, there is another side to this drug: it can cause cancer of the nose, which Freud developed and died from, and it can erode the cartilage between the nostrils so that there is no visible partition between them, which is cosmetically very unattractive. In high doses it can cause death from seizures, heart attacks and suppression of the breathing centre in the brain.

Addiction

It is a highly addictive drug and because it produces such a positive feeling of well-being a psychological dependence can develop after a single use. In addition, increasing doses are required to achieve the desired effect and profound depression is common during withdrawal. The effects of snorting cocaine are felt almost immediately but are relatively brief in duration, wearing off after thirty to sixty minutes. Colleagues at work often notice that the cocaine addict has to excuse themselves every thirty minutes or so to go to a secluded spot to snort cocaine.

Personality Change

Perhaps you have noticed that your friends who take cocaine are very changeable in personality. In particular, irritability and poor concentration become noticeable in users. Anxiety, panic attacks and repetitive behaviours such as checking, touching objects and so on are common also. Cocaine affects mood by increasing well-being, but it is followed by severe depression (known as a crash) and suicidal thoughts, and sometimes attempts, during withdrawal.

It becomes increasingly difficult for users to function at work. Nasal congestion results in altered speech. Energy levels are increased and so the person who has taken cocaine over-estimates their capacity to perform. This leads to severe insomnia and exhaustion. Cocaine is used as an aphrodisiac and to delay orgasm, but repeated use can lead to impotence.

Mini-strokes

Cocaine can cause brain damage, not due to the direct toxic effect on the brain cells, as with other drugs such as "ecstasy", but due to mini-strokes and clots, which impair the oxygen supply. Epileptic fits occur in cocaine abusers and sometimes these can be prolonged. Those who take "crack" or who use large amounts of cocaine are most at risk. Cocaine and "crack" can also cause heart attacks and an irregular heart beat.

Reality

Loss of touch with reality is probably the most dangerous and worrying aspect of cocaine addiction due to its very high frequency, affecting about 50 per cent of users. In particular, the belief that others are persecuting the individual can lead to aggression and homicidal or other violent behaviour. Sometimes users frequently describe a feeling of insects crawling under the skin. There may also be visual hallucination with the user hearing voices that are not actually present.

* * *

You can see that, fashionable though cocaine and crack-cocaine may be, these are highly dangerous substances. I suggest you find other outlets and other friends. These people are being foolish and naive and you are wise to be very cautious indeed. Cocaine is not safe for recreational use; it is highly dangerous.

Useful Website

www.nlm.nih.gov/medlineplus/cocaineabuse.html

Useful Contact

Trinity Court
Pierce Street, Dublin 2, Tel. (01) 6770122

I work as a teacher and during a recent discussion with the Leaving Cert class I realised that many of them seemed to think that there was no danger associated with taking ecstasy. Is it possible that some of them are taking it very regularly? They seemed to have good knowledge of it – or perhaps it was just bravado. I know that there have been several deaths associated with it in Britain but I know very little else about it. Can you give me more information?

Ecstasy is known as a designer drug, as it is synthesised from pre-existing synthetic drugs known as amphetamines. Surprisingly, ecstasy was first made in 1912 as an appetite suppressant but rapidly fell out of use until the 1970s, when it was used by some psychotherapists in the United States because of its ability to induce empathic feelings for others and to release emotion. This use was controversial and little was heard of it until the early 1990s, when it became popular as a drug of recreational use at rock-concerts and late-night parties called "raves".

Endurance Drug

Ecstasy now embraces a wide range of similar drugs, all chemically related to amphetamines, but the best-known one is MDMA. It is taken in tablet, capsule or powder form and costs a few pounds – relatively cheap. Most of the drug is manufactured in illegal laboratories in Western Europe, with a smaller amount coming from the United States.

The immediate effects include an increase in energy, extreme relaxation, a positive feeling for oneself and for others and the elimination of tension and worry. In addition, it suppresses the need to eat, drink or sleep so that it is possible to endure parties lasting several days. It is for this reason that it is so popular and if your pupils are regular attenders at all-night parties it is certainly possible that they may be taking "E". Because thirst and tiredness are eliminated there is a danger of severe dehydration and exhaustion, resulting in heart failure and death.

Effects on Users

Some users experience hallucinations, increases in body temperature, blurred vision and muscle cramps. When body temperature rises, a problem most likely to occur after several tablets have been consumed, water is drunk in large quantities and there is a danger of water intoxication or heat stroke, resulting in death. It was in these circumstances that the deaths you mention occurred. Some users develop a psychosis with hallucinations (seeing and hearing things that are not there) and disorientation but these subside in a few days. At times they may require admission to hospital to treat these symptoms. Feelings of being cut-off, of being outside oneself, can also occur and last for several days. These are very frightening.

Perhaps you have noticed a cycle of mood changes among the pupils who may be using this drug. Taken on its own, the user will feel relaxed and contented for a day or so afterwards. However, this does not last and by the end of the second day, mood is low and irritability is noticeable. This continues for about two days and by day five mood and behaviour are back to normal. So even those who take it only at weekends are at risk of being almost continually affected. Indeed, some try to improve their low mood on days three and four by taking extra, thereby lengthening the period of depression rather than shortening it, since the cycle begins again.

Brain Damage

Only recently have the long-term effects begun to be studied. Preliminary findings are worrying, as they show that regular use is associated with damage to the nerves in the brain that transmit a chemical called serotonin. This is involved in a number of functions including the modulation of emotions, learning and sleep. If these findings are correct then regular recreational users are at risk of permanent brain damage manifesting itself as depression, memory loss and anxiety.

* * *

Contrary to what some of your pupils say, "E" is associated with serious short- and long-term problems that are just coming to light. It is worth bearing in mind that its sister drug, amphetamine, was first made in 1887 and was licensed for use by doctors in the 1930s. Not until the late 1960s were the problems associated with amphetamines officially accepted. The story of amphetamines should be a lesson to us all.

Useful Website

www.nida.nih.gov/DrugAbuse.html
(Click on MDMA)

Useful Contact

Trinity Court
Pierce Street, Dublin 2, Tel. (01) 6770122

I have just been told that my brother has a condition called an "amphetamine psychosis". He has been taking drugs for some time and about two weeks ago he began to act strangely. This resulted in his admission to a psychiatric unit. He is much improved now but has been warned never to take drugs again. I take drugs occasionally also and I don't see any harm in them, for me. I think this is just scaremongering.

I am glad that your brother is improving but as you will appreciate he has had a serious condition and it is one that may recur and become more serious. It is essential that he refrain from ever abusing drugs again.

Medical Use

Amphetamines, as you probably know, are known on the street as "speed" and "crystal". They have been available since first being synthesised in 1887 and have been in medical use since the 1930s. They were easily available for a variety of medical disorders until the 1970s, when their abuse became a problem. Following legal control they are now only legally dispensed for use, in this country, for the treatment of attention deficit hyperactivity disorder (ADHD) in children and adolescents. When used in the treatment of this disorder, amphetamines tend not to cause the problems that are associated with their abuse such as you have described.

Energising

Amphetamines can be inhaled, taken by mouth or injected intravenously and their effects are rapid in onset and very powerful, often described as "whole body orgasm". When consumed orally the effect occurs within one hour; when injected intravenously, the effect is immediate. The speed of onset is one of the reasons for their popularity as well as the actual pleasurable effects they produce.

They are used by those who want to improve performance – students studying for exams, athletes in competitions and business people who need to meet deadlines. In small doses they can induce elation and a sense of wellbeing and friendliness; they can improve concentration and performance and reduce tiredness. They are also used as "uppers" to counteract the profound lowering of mood during withdrawal from cocaine or heroin, known as "downers", although when amphetamines themselves are stopped mood can also plunge into gloom.

Psychotic Reactions

Although amphetamines provide energy and are sought after by many, they have serious psychiatric effects that are often not discussed. It is important that you get to know a little bit about these so as to inform yourself and your brother. Loss of touch with reality taking the form of hallucinations and delusions, especially that you are being persecuted, is the most serious. This is known as amphetamine psychosis, the condition that your brother had. There is also incoherence of speech and visual hallucinations (seeing things that are not actually present). Amphetamine psychosis generally clears up within seven days. However, there is evidence that in some vulnerable people it can progress to schizophrenia and this would be a worry with your brother. Other less serious disturbances include lowering of mood, impotence, insomnia and anxiety disorders.

Caution

It is likely that your brother will make a full recovery, but if he continues to abuse this or other mind-altering drugs he may and probably will have a recurrence and might ultimately go on to develop schizophrenia. As you are his sister, you too may have the same vulnerability to these reactions to amphetamines and you should also avoid them – there is no definitive test that can confirm or disprove your predisposition to similar reactions. This is not scare mongering, but is based on research and on my own practice where amphetamines often trigger schizophrenia.

* * *

Your brother can remain well and you would greatly assist him in this if you too remained drug free. You should encourage him to accept all the professional help that is available and to remain on his prescribed medication. There is no soft option for your brother, or for you. You should not take amphetamines.

Useful Website

www.nida.nih.gov/DrugAbuse.html
(Click on methamphetaime)

Useful Contact

Drug Treatment Centre
30/31 Pearse Street, Dublin 2, Tel. (01) 6771122

I recently saw my brother withdrawing from heroin. I have been trying to persuade him to get help for his problem but he is so reluctant. The withdrawal was terrifying for us all. He was vomiting and in a lot of discomfort. He just sat it out for a few days but I never want to see it happen again. Is this usual?

You are correct when you say that heroin withdrawal is frightening – it certainly is, for the person experiencing it as well as for those who witness it. Heroin is an opiate and belongs to the same group of drugs as morphine and pethidine, drugs that are used when severe pain is present such as in cancer, during childbirth or after major surgery. Heroin is not available for general medical use and is only used by addicts.

Cold Turkey

These drugs should not be given continuously for more than a few weeks as dependence occurs and then withdrawal reactions follow their discontinuation. Coming off opiates is known as "kicking cold turkey" and this is what your brother did.

Risks

Heroin is the most addictive drug of all the opiates, since it is the most potent and it rapidly induces feelings of euphoria and contentment. However, there are complications with the use of any opiate including the risk of death due to suppression of the breathing centre in the brain. If these drugs are injected, using shared needles, there is the risk of hepatitis and HIV.

Withdrawal

Although your brother seems to have had just a few symptoms, there are other withdrawal symptoms such as nausea, watery eyes, constant yawning, high temperature, aches and pains, diarrhoea, low mood and dilated pupils that make the withdrawal very distressing indeed.

Although heroin induces euphoria when taken initially, with time this lessens and the amount taken has to be increased to achieve a continuing effect – this is known as tolerance. Sometimes an addict just takes drugs to prevent the unpleasant withdrawal symptoms. These begin within six to eight hours of the last dose, reach a peak in two or three days and subside after about seven days. The withdrawal, although uncomfortable is generally not life threatening.

Nowadays there is no need for anybody to have to go through "cold turkey" as did your brother, since there are established treatment clinics in our cities.

Detoxify

The ideal is to gradually detoxify the person who is addicted and maintain them in a drug-free state. This may require a period of in-patient treatment using a related drug called methadone. Heroin is replaced with methadone and the dose is decreased over a period of a few weeks. If your brother had sought professional help this is the approach that would almost certainly have been adopted. However, it is not always possible to remain drug free and so maintenance methadone is prescribed in special clinics under strict supervision. The purpose of this is to remove the addict from the black market and gain some control over the amount of opiate being consumed.

Methadone

Although methadone is itself an opiate and is therefore addictive, it is less so than heroin because it does not cause the intense pleasurable feeling or "rush" that heroin does. The withdrawal symptoms from methadone are milder than those of heroin.

Sometimes in methadone clinics free needles are also exchanged to reduce the need for dirty needles and ultimately the risk of serious infection. Since high levels of commitment to kick the habit are required, to help motivation some centres use a drug called naltrexone to block the pleasurable effects of these opiates.

Counselling

As well as these chemical treatments, counselling is used to assist in maintaining motivation and to address other background problems that the addict may have. Some addicts benefit from a stay in a residential unit for a few months. Above all, the two most important factors in successfully combating these drugs are support from family and friends and the motivation to persist.

* * *

From what you say, your brother certainly seems to have the support of yourself and hopefully of other family members also. Let us hope that he has the desire to remain drug free.

Useful Reading

Kenny, M. (1999) *Death by Heroin: Recovery by Hope*, New Island Books: Dublin

Useful Website

www.nida.nih.gov/DrugAbuse.html
(Click on opiates)

Useful Contact

Drug Treatment Centre
30–31 Trinity Court, Pearse Street, Dublin 2, Tel. (01) 6771122

Suicide

There is but one truly serious philosophical problem, and that is suicide. Judging whether life is or is not worth living amounts to answering the fundamental question of philosophy.

Albert Camus,
"An Absurd Reasoning", The Myth of Sisyphus, *trans. 1955*

I have a twenty-three-year-old daughter and recently she has become a bit quieter than usual. She had a boyfriend for the past six months but she broke up with him recently and told me she was relieved, as he was possessive. Her work is going well and she has a small group of very close friends. She told me recently she was a bit fed up and that sometimes she feels she would be better off dead. I am absolutely terrified that she is suicidal. What can I do without being an alarmist?

It is unusual for somebody so young to feel so gloomy and down, particularly when there is no particular reason in her personal or professional life. As you say her life seems to be going well at present in spite of the recent break-up with her boyfriend. It is important that you try to talk with her and since you seem to have a close relationship with her, she may well speak freely with you. In particular, you are concerned that she may be suicidal. Many people use phrases such as "better off dead" on the spur of the moment. It is possible that it was in this way she was using the term and if so, then it was a throwaway remark that is not likely to be associated with suicidal thoughts.

Take it Seriously

However, you indicate that she has not been her old self recently and coupled with this remark the change you describe must be taken seriously. When you speak with her you must find out what she meant by her comment and if she really does feel that she would be better off dead, even for a brief period. You could ask, "You said recently that you feel you might be better of dead. Did you mean this or was it just a chance remark?" You should also ask if she means that she would like to go to sleep and not wake up or if she had something else in mind? Many people just want to go to sleep but wouldn't dream of harming themselves. This is known as a passive death wish and whilst it can sometimes herald later suicidal ideas, of itself it is not associated with suicidal behaviour.

If your daughter tells you that she had something more than just going to sleep in mind then you should try to find out if she has plans to harm herself and how clearly formed they are. In all probability you will not feel comfortable asking these types of questions and indeed she may be embarrassed talking to you about such personal matters.

Professional Help

You should encourage your daughter to visit her general practitioner. If she is reluctant to follow your advice she may accept the advice of a friend or somebody outside the family whom she trusts. Whilst you may be reluctant to interfere in your adult daughter's life, it would be no harm to alert the general practitioner to the fact that you are worried about what she has been saying to you and about the recent observed change, at the same time as assuring the doctor that you absolutely respect your daughter's right to confidentiality.

Undoubtedly, this will be of great assistance to the doctor, who will want to ascertain if she is suicidal and, if she is, what is causing her present state of mind. Even if she is not suicidal, the doctor will want to find out why her spirits are low – is it because of problems that she may not have told you about or does she have a clinical depression? She would then need further psychological/psychiatric help.

Clinical Depression

Clinical depression can occur with or without a background stressor and it could certainly account for the change you see in her as well as for the things she has said to you. If she does have clinical depression her doctor may wish to prescribe antidepressants. These are very effective and can bring about improvement in a few weeks. Thereafter further psychotherapy may also be required. If your daughter is suicidal, urgent referral to a psychiatrist may be necessary also. On no account must you accept promises from her such as "Oh, don't worry about me, I'll be OK, I'm just run down" or some such explanation.

* * *

Doing nothing could be the worst thing, so please sit down and listen to what she tells you as well as offering your full support.

Useful Reading

Golant, M. and Golant, S.K. (1998) *What to Do When Someone You Love Is Depressed*, Owl Books: New York

Useful Website

www.nami.org/helpline/suicide.htm

Useful Contact

AWARE
72 Lower Leeson Street, Dublin 2, Tel. (01) 6617211

I think my brother may be suicidal. He is thirty-five and has become very quiet in the past few months. He isn't going out at all although he was very sociable before this. I took some comfort from the fact that he said he felt like killing himself, as I understand that those who talk about it don't do it. Do you think he needs to have tests to find out why he is feeling like this?

Your brother most definitely needs to see a doctor and I would say that should happen as soon as possible. One of the myths about suicide is that those who talk about it do not act on their urges. This is incorrect: the fact that he is talking about it should alert you to the distress that he is experiencing.

Talking and Listening

Apart from ruling out physical conditions, such as disease of the thyroid gland or alcohol abuse, as causes of low mood, there is no blood test or psychological test to help in this. The only way is to speak with your brother in a non-threatening, non-confrontational way and explore what he is thinking in this regard. For example, does he have continuing thoughts of self-harm? What plans, if any, does he have? When and where does he intend harming himself? Sometimes those who are suicidal give subtle warnings such as contacting old friends, making a will or taking out an insurance policy. It would also be crucial to examine his reasons for not harming himself. These might include his family, his hope that things will get better and religious beliefs. In many it is the balance between the reasons for living or for dying that sustains the depressed person and stops them ending their life.

Asking the Question

You may be surprised to be advised to talk to your brother about suicidal thoughts but one of the other myths is that asking about suicide will plant the idea in the person's mind. There is no evidence to suggest that raising the question stimulates suicide – after all, your brother has raised the issue with you. It must of course be done gently and sensitively, but with the awareness that sometimes those who are suicidal will conceal their intentions so that they can carry out their plan. You should be very watchful if, for example, your brother has been agitated and perplexed and then becomes calm, as this may be an indication that he has made a definite decision about ending his life. You must also bear in mind that if he has ever harmed himself or overdosed in the past then the risk is much higher.

Contact your Doctor

You will probably feel uncomfortable talking with him in this way and your doctor is the obvious person to do this. If your brother refuses to visit the doctor then perhaps his wife (if he is married) or some other person to whom he is close and respects might prevail upon him. If that still fails then you would be justified in contacting the doctor yourself and asking their advice on how to proceed.

Offering Help

Once your brother has visited the doctor the help that will be offered depends on how depressed your brother is and, more especially, whether the doctor thinks he is suicidal. If your brother is harbouring serious suicidal plans then the doctor would want him seen by a psychiatrist urgently, which might result in him being admitted to hospital for an assessment. If, however, the thoughts were fleeting and have now passed then the doctor might feel it more appropriate to treat him himself. If your brother has a depressive illness that is causing the suicidal thoughts then medication may be required; if your brother is under stress due to some life problem the doctor may refer him for counselling.

* * *

Ultimately, it is important for you to realise that suicidal thoughts must always be investigated and that in most instances the causes of these can be addressed.

Useful Reading

Golant, M. and Golant, S.K. (1998) *What to Do when Someone you Love Is Depressed*, Owl Books: New York

Useful Website

www.nami.org/helpline/suicide.htm

I am forty-seven and I have been reading a lot about suicide recently. I sometimes feel so hopeless and helpless that I think I would be better off dead. I have no particular problems except that I worry about my children's future. My husband and I have a good marriage and I also enjoyed working outside the home until recently. Now it is just such a hassle that I feel like giving it up. Part of me does not want to die; I just want peace of mind and contentment restored again.

It is unusual to feel so gloomy and down, especially when there is no particular problem in your family or professional life. It sounds as though your concern about your children is a general one and I suspect it is no different from the natural concerns that all parents have. Your concern might also be related to your low mood, since how we feel in ourselves can distort our view of the world and of those around us.

Unburdening

One positive thing is that you have a good relationship with your husband so if you unburden yourself to him it may be of some benefit, although he is not a professional and it would be unfair to expect him to become your therapist. You may also want to talk with a friend or a priest. Ultimately, if the feelings of sadness and gloom persist you will need professional help.

"I Need Help"

Many people speak of wanting to die as a casual, almost throwaway remark, when in reality they have no intention of taking any action to this end. This phrase is often a way of saying "I feel sad. I need help". When you get these thoughts is it really true that you believe the only way out is to take your life? During your happier moments you should ask yourself the same question: "Is suicide the only solution?" "Would my family be better off without me if I took my own life?" The fact that part of you does not really want to die suggests that deep down you know that your family cares for you and that they would be devastated if you did die by suicide, or indeed from any illness. When you ask yourself these questions you should also write down the answer and carry it with you. It could serve as a reminder to you that your view of the world and the future is distorted during these bleak moments. Therefore, major decisions about any matter, least of all about life and death, should not be made in that state.

Professional Help

You indicate that in other respects, such as in work, you have not been your old self. I suggest that you visit your doctor and talk to them openly about your difficulties, feelings and symptoms. For example, what is your confidence like at present? How are you sleeping? Have you lost weight? Have your interests declined? Have you slowed down at work? Sometimes concentration may be very poor so that mistakes are made in relation to money and so on.

Some of the things you mention in the letter suggest that you may have a clinical depression, often referred to as depressive illness. This illness can occur with or without a background stressor so it is not impossible for somebody like you whose life is good in all respects to develop this disorder. If you do have clinical depression your general practitioner may wish to prescribe antidepressants. These are very effective and can bring about improvement in a few weeks. If you ever become suicidal and begin to make plans to end your life, an immediate assessment by a psychiatrist may be necessary.

* * *

Doing nothing could be the worst thing, so please sit down and talk with your husband, since his full support will be necessary. Also, do not delay going to your general practitioner – in a short while you will begin to see that life is worth going on with and you will be back to your old self again.

Useful Website

www.nami.org/helpline/suicide.htm

Useful Contact

AWARE
72 Lower Leeson Street, Dublin 2, Tel. (01) 6617211

I often feel suicidal and I have thought of harming myself. On a few occasions I actually made a definite plan but seeing my wife and child stopped me. This has been happening for the past two years since my mother took her own life, although she had been depressed for many years and refused help. I feel so guilty because everything is going well for me. I have a good job and my wife and I love each other deeply and I don't want to worry her. I am terrified of going to my general practitioner.

I am sure it must be dreadful for you to feel so low that you feel like ending your life. Many people experience passing thoughts like this from time to time but what worries me about what you have told me is that these thoughts seem to be recurring and you even made plans to harm yourself.

Getting Help

You must get professional help and I strongly recommend you see your general practitioner. They may be able to find a cause or suggest that you see a specialist. Contrary to popular perception, people are not locked up any more. In fact, most of the help that people need can be obtained by attending the out-patient clinic. Sometimes when a person has active suicidal plans and is at serious risk of carrying them out at that time, admission may be required. This is usually for a short period until the cause has been identified and the person is beginning to deal with the underlying problem or is able to distance themselves enough from their predicament.

We all need confidants, especially for our most painful thoughts. At present you need somebody too. I can understand that you may not wish to worry your wife but your marriage seems very stable. You should tell her how you feel. If you cannot tell your wife, you must confide in somebody. I suggest a friend, priest, general practitioner or family member.

Searching for the Problem

Often when people feel very low they look to the past to try to find something there to explain this. In your case, you say there is nothing but you have had major trauma in your life with your mother's tragic death and also her depression. Parental depression can have an effect on a young person growing up. Since your mother had depression it is crucial that this be explored further with you – the possibility that you may have depression must be examined, as it can sometimes be masked behind various other symptoms such as lack of sleep, lack up concentration and appetite changes.

Acknowledge your Problem

From what you have said in your letter it is clear that you recognise that you may have a psychological problem; you have a good life yet you contemplate suicide. The fact that you have asked me for advice shows that you know that your present emotional state and your suicidal thoughts are not based on your real life circumstances but on how you are feeling.

* * *

No matter how you are feeling at present I urge you to please read the book suggested below in order to get a perspective on your situation. You must also contact your doctor whom I am sure will be of great help to you. If you feel you cannot, then talk with the Samaritans who will hear your story and be there to listen to your sadness. However, you do need medical help just now.

Useful Reading

Golant, M. and Golant, S.K. (1998) *What to Do when Someone you Love Is Depressed*, Owl Books: New York

Useful Website

www.nami.org/helpline/suicide.htm

Useful Contacts

AWARE
72 Lower Leeson Street, Dublin 2, Tel. (01) 6617211

The Samaritans
Tel. (01) 8727700

My seventeen-year-old daughter recently attempted suicide by taking an overdose of seven paracetamol tablets. She took them from the medicine cabinet following a row about being out late. She didn't leave any suicide note and came to the bedroom to tell us about it immediately. We took her to the A&E where she was pumped out and seen by a psychiatrist. He said she had no psychiatric disorder – but surely she must have to do such a thing.

I am sorry that you have had this trauma to deal with. Unfortunately, there are many young people nowadays who take overdoses in similar circumstances to those of your daughter. These acts are mainly done on impulse. Unlike an act that is truly an attempt at suicide, these are not planned and are more a gesture of anger or defiance than an attempt to end life. Calling them suicide attempts is therefore not an accurate description of what motivates them.

The terms parasuicide (paralleling suicide) and deliberate self-harm are words used by professionals to describe these self-destructive behaviours such as you describe. Within this totality there are a very small proportion of people who are truly trying to take their life. The remainder are like your daughter – acting out of anger or else using their behaviour as a way of getting help for their problems. This has been called the "cry for help" phenomenon and although often talked about it is not very common.

Assessment

The reason your daughter was seen by a psychiatrist in the A&E department was to evaluate her mood and assess any psychological problems that might require help. So the psychiatrist was assessing whether she had a clinical depression or another disorder that required specific treatment, or any particular social or personal problems that would benefit from the help of either a psychologist or psychiatrist. Most importantly he was assessing whether she was still suicidal at the time she was seen. The fact that she was allowed home suggests that she was no longer having self-destructive thoughts and that she did not have any specific psychiatric disorder or any particular problems requiring immediate professional help. If you are still worried about your daughter or you feel that some problems were not mentioned in the assessment you could speak with the family doctor, who is in the best position to advise you if further help is required.

Low Suicide Risk

You are understandably very worried that your daughter might kill herself in the future. About 1 per cent of those who self-harm go on to eventually take their lives during the subsequent year. These are people who repeatedly self-harm or who have psychiatric disorders such as untreated or severe clinical depression or chronic alcohol abuse. So the probability of this happening is low. However, suicide is always very difficult to predict, even in those with serious psychiatric disorder, since it is a rare, albeit tragic, event.

Professional Help

It would seem that your daughter's behaviour, although potentially dangerous, is a reflection of her difficulty coping with conflict. You can take comfort from the fact that she does not have an identifiable psychiatric illness at present. You should also realise that as your daughter matures she will learn more appropriate responses to personal difficulties. If she wishes she could seek the help of a clinical psychologist, who would help her discover more suitable problem-solving skills than those she has at present. Most important, however, is that she rebuilds her relationship with you. If there are continuing difficulties between you, you might think of family therapy – this would involve several meetings between the family, including your daughter, and a trained therapist who would identify the problems that are arising and assist you in resolving them before they get out of hand.

* * *

I hope that you and your daughter resolve your difficulties.

Useful Reading

Butler, Gillian and Hope, Tony (1998) *Manage Your Mind: The Mental Fitness Guide*, Oxford University Press: Oxford

Useful Contact

AWARE
72 Lower Leeson Street, Dublin 2, Tel. (01) 6617211

I live in a village where there have recently been several suicides within a period of a few months. Unfortunately, all the people concerned knew each other, although they were not close friends. I am very surprised by this as I have always heard that suicide was associated with psychiatric illness such as depression or alcoholism yet these young people did not have any problems that I know of. The whole community is deeply shocked and thinks this may be an example of "copy-cat" suicide.

Sadly, your story is very common and, like you, communities feel bewildered and helpless.

"Werther Effect"

Copy-cat suicide is termed the "Werther Effect" after a character in a book *The Sorrows of Young Werther* by Goethe. Unfortunately, many people do not realise that suicide is "infectious" and that there is a contagion effect. In the United States research shows that the under twenty-five age group are especially susceptible to this, although it is only in recent years that this has been recognised.

Some years ago a German television station broadcast a play about a young person taking his life. A psychiatrist named Schmitke studied the suicide trends thereafter and found that there was a rise in the subsequent six months with a levelling off after that. This was dismissed as coincidence at that time. However, several years later the play was broadcast again and the same investigator repeated his study and found the same result. It is now well-recognised that suicide is sometimes imitated.

Coverage

It is undoubtedly true that high-profile cases such as the suicide of Kurt Cobain receive unprecedented media attention. As such people are often role models, in a variety of ways, the attention directed to their death may influence young people, especially those that closely identify with the person, to follow this example. For this reason the media must be very careful about the manner in which the death is reported and should not give details of the method or place. However, even with ordinary people, there is now evidence that detailed coverage of the manner of their deaths such as publishing details of the inquest may be associated with additional suicides.

An issue that is increasingly being investigated is whether it is the manner of reporting a suicide death that triggers further suicides or if the simple fact of reporting the death by suicide is associated with this contagion. If this were true then even general discussion about suicide might carry a risk.

There are some studies to suggest that prevention programmes in schools, such as general talks about how to recognise a suicidal friend or colleague, might trigger suicide in the vulnerable by normalising it. It is not that every teenager is likely to be put at risk, but those in whom suicidal ideas might be evolving are likely to be in danger. The work of Shaffer from Columbia University is exploring this aspect of the suicide problem at present.

Community Response

I am sure that your community finds it hard to know what to do in these circumstances. Of course, you must be there to support the family of the deceased and if they need to talk about their loss with you then you must of course facilitate this. Also, if you know of anybody who may be depressed, you or a friend should encourage that person to seek professional help.

It is vital that suicide not be glorified and it must be named for what it is – a devastating blow to a family that brings untold suffering. In addition discussions about whether it is a noble or a cowardly act have no place: it is neither – it is an act of hopelessness and desperation. No blame must attach to anybody, least of all the family, as they will undoubtedly be blaming themselves.

It is common for communities to try to respond to suicides by attempting to understand suicide itself. On the face of it this might seem a good idea. However, great care needs to be exercised about any public meeting in view of the potential for the discussion of suicide to act as a trigger, especially if there is any possibility that it could be glorified.

* * *

You and your community have my greatest sympathy and there is no simple, certain or easy way for you all to heal your grief. Being there in a personal way for those who need to talk about it is itself remarkable in the comfort it can bring.

Useful Reading

Jamison, Kay Redfield (2000) *Night Falls Fast*, Vintage Books: New York

Useful Website

www.nami.org/helpline/suicide.htm

Useful Contact

The Samaritans
Tel. (01) 8727700

Index

AA (Alcoholics Anonymous) 244, 251
abnormal stress 231–232, 238–239
   normal versus 231–232
abortion, bereavement after 51–52
acamprosate 244
agoraphobia 13–15, 22
   panic attacks and 14, 22
Al-anon 244
alcohol
   effects on depression 87
   insomnia and 109
   undesirable effects 243
alcohol abuse 155, 243–252
   brain damage 61, 65
   building tolerance 243
   colluding with heavy drinker 248
   complications 251
   depression and 250
   drying out (detoxification) 243, 250–251
   effects on children 248
   help needed for 244
   secrecy of 249
   treatment 244
alcoholic dementia 61
alcoholics
   accepting drink problem 248–249
   compulsory treatment 123, 244, 246
alexythymia 143
alternative medicines 3–4
alternative therapies 1–9
   hypnotherapy 7–9
   Omega-3 oil 4
   St John's Wort 3–4, 5–6

Alzheimer's disease 61, 64, 65, 206
   memory enhancers 60
   validity of will made by sufferer 125–126
   vascular dementia and 59, 60
amphetamines 255, 257, 258, 259–260
   amphetamine psychosis 259–260
   psychotic reactions 260
anorexia nervosa 103–104
   advice for parents 103
   professional help 103–104
   treatment 104
antabuse 251
antidepressants 19, 236, 250
   breastfeeding and 96
   counselling versus 72
   post-natal depression and 96–97
   for premenstrual syndrome (PMS) 188
   safety information 97
   side effects 71–72
   SSRIs 71, 75, 96, 188
   and tranquillizers 71
   tricyclic antidepressants 71
antisocial behaviour 162, 163
anxiety
   feigning 129–130
   psychiatric services for 170–171
   reducing levels 19
anxiety disorders 11–39
   agoraphobia 13–15, 22
   cat phobia 31–33
   debriefing 38–39
   depersonalisation 20–21
   derealisation 20–21

anxiety disorders—*contd.*
  generalised anxiety 18
  obsessive-compulsive disorder 24–25, 26–27
  panic attacks 22–23
  panic disorder 22
  relaxation tapes for 36
  social anxiety 28–30
  tranquillizers for 16–17, 34–35, 36–37
  worrying 18–19, 36–37
asylum seekers and refugees, emotional problems 143–145
attention deficit hyperactivity disorder (ADHD) 137–138, 259
  diagnosis 137
  treatment 138, 259
  types 137–138

behaviour therapy 13, 27, 32, 156, 215
bereavement 41–55
  after suicide 47–48, 53–55
  anger and 47
  coming to terms with 43
  crying 43, 45, 46
  following abortion 51–52
  following miscarriage 49–50
  healing 43–44, 48
  looking at photographs 45–46
  mixed emotions 46, 53
  professional help 44
  reminders 45–46
  visiting the grave 43, 45
bereavement counselling 44, 45
bipolar disorder *see* manic-depression
borderline personality disorder 155–157
  diagnosis 155, 156
  improvement from 155–156
  symptoms 155
  treatment 156
bulimia nervosa 105–106
  coping with food anxieties 105
  getting help from family 105–106
  reward system 106

cannabis 253–254
  cannabis psychosis 253
  effects 253–254
  psychological dependence 254
carbamazepine 83
cat phobia 31–33
  avoiding cats 31
  behaviour therapy 32
  exposure sessions 32
  self-help 31–32
certification, to psychiatric units 123–124, 246–247
children, custody battles 121–122
clinical depression 69–70, 268, 272
  effects of pleasant events 69
  prevalence 69–70
  sexual abuse and 198
  stress reactions and 234–235
  symptoms 69, 236
  treatment of 70
  see also depression, depressive illness
cocaine 255–256
  addiction 255
  effects of 255, 256
  personality changes 255–256
cognitive therapy 29, 72, 78, 80–81, 104, 182–184, 215
  cognitions 182
  counselling and 183
  techniques 182–183
compulsory admission to psychiatric hospital 123–124, 246–247
  grounds for 123, 246
  legislation 247
  process 123–124, 246
confabulations 61–62
conversion disorder 129
copy-cat suicide 277–279
counselling 29, 72, 183, 214, 235, 262
court reports 119–120
crimes, committed by person with serious mental illness 131–133
criminals, protecting public from mentally ill 132

Index

Critical Incident Stress Debriefing 38
"cry for help" phenomenon 275
custody battles
   deciding best arrangement for children 121
   depression and 122
   going to court 122
   independent assessment 121

debriefing 38–39, 215
defence mechanisms 180
delirium tremens (the DTs) 250
delusions 207
dementia 57–65
   alcoholic dementia 61
   atherosclerotic dementia 65
   frontal lobe dementia 62
   multi-infarct dementia 59–60
   pseudodementia 64
   vascular dementia 59–60
depersonalisation 20, 21, 34
   causes 20–21
   specialist treatment 21
depression 4, 18
   alcohol and 87, 250
   causative factors 89–90
   custody battles and 122
   dysthymia 77, 78
   endogenous (spontaneous) depression 77–79, 90
   erectile dysfunction and 193
   feigning 129–130
   inheritance of 92–93
   insomnia in 112
   manic-depression 4, 78, 80–81, 82–84, 92, 155, 172
   masked depression 112
   memory loss and 64
   menopause and 189
   post-natal depression 78, 93, 94–95, 96–97
   protection from 90
   in psychiatrist's report 119–120
   reactive depression 77
   reading about 85–86

depression—*contd.*
   recurrence 73
   recurrent depressive disorder 78
   returning to activities after 85, 87–88
   risk factors 89, 90
   seasonal affective disorder (SAD) 78, 98–99
   Seroxat drug treatment 75–76
   sleep rhythm 87
   steroids and 146–147
   St John's Wort and 5–6
   stress and recovery 86
   support from loved ones 74
   support groups 86
   treatment 73, 78
   types of 77–79
   see also clinical depression, depressive illness
depressive illness 18, 19, 71–72, 92–93, 272
   antidepressants 71–72
   cognitive therapy 183
   counselling treatment 72
   shoplifting and 127
   symptoms 69
   triggers 234, 235
   vulnerability 235
   see also clinical depression, depression
derealisation 20, 21, 34
dissociative identity disorder 158–159
disulfiram 244, 251
doctors, confidentiality adherence 174–175
double blind theory 211
drug addiction 226, 255, 256, 261–262
dyspareunia 195
dysthymia 77, 78

eating disorders 101–106
   anorexia nervosa 103–104
   bulimia nervosa 105–106
ecstasy 257–258
elation, steroid side effect 147

"empty nest" syndrome 190
erectile dysfunction 193–194

false memory syndrome 8
family schism and skew 211
family therapy 104, 215, 276
forgetfulness 64, 65, 127, 223
frontal lobe dementia 62

Ganser syndrome 129
grieving 43–44, 46, 47, 48, 143–144

heroin 261–263
   counselling for addicts 262
   detoxification 262
   methadone and 262
   risks 261
   withdrawal symptoms 261
homosexuality 191–192
   causes 192
   myths 191
hospital addiction 225
HRT 189, 190
hypericum 5, 6
hypersomnia 112
hypnosis 7–9
   dangers of 8
   hypnotic induction 7–8
   suggestibility 8
   uses of 7
hysteria 129

impotence 193–194
   causes of 193–194
   investigations 194
   prevalence 193
   treatment 194
insomnia 107–113, 146
   causes of 109
   in depression 112
   hypersomnia 112
   lifestyle habits 109–110
   management of 110, 113
   medication 110
   symptoms 112

jealousy, in relationships 139–140

khat 144
kleptomania 127, 128
Korsakoff's psychosis 61

lamotrigine 83
libido, loss of 195–196
lithium 4, 78, 80, 82–84

malingering 129–130, 223–224
   confronting malingerer 224
   fooling doctors 224
   symptoms 223
manic-depression 4, 78, 80–81, 82–84, 92, 155
   bipolar 1 80
   bipolar 2 80
   forms 80
   lithium treatment 4, 78, 80, 82–84
   psychiatric services 172–173
   treatment 80–81, 82–83
marriage annulment 117–118, 162
   grounds for 117, 162
   legal advice 118
   personality factors 117–118
medico-legal issues 115–133
   compulsory admission to psychiatric hospital 123–124
   crimes committed by person with serious mental illness 131–133
   custody battles for children 121–122
   feigning psychiatric illness 129–130
   marriage annulment 117–118
   psychiatrist's report 119–120
   shoplifting 127–128
   validity of wills 125–126
melancholia 5
memory loss 64–65
   causes of 64–65
   dealing with 65
menopause 70, 189–190
   depressive illness and 189
   male menopause 190
   myths 189–190

Index 285

methadone 262
miscarriage, grieving after 49–50
M'Naghten's Rules 131–132
multiple personality disorder
   158–159
   diagnosis 158–159
   legal implications 159
   main features 158
Munchausen's by Proxy 226
Munchausen's syndrome 225–227
   feigning symptoms 225
   motivation 225–226
   treatment 226

naltrexone 262
nervous breakdown 85

obsessional personality disorder
   162–163
obsessive-compulsive disorder (OCD)
   24–25, 26–27
   progress in understanding 26
   self-help 25
   treatment 26, 27
Omega-3 oil 4
Othello syndrome 140
Out and About organisation 13
overdosing 155, 156, 275–276

panic attacks 18, 22–23
   agoraphobia and 14
   diary of symptoms 23
   therapy 22–23
panic disorder 22
paranoid psychosis 205–206
   causes 205–206
   diagnosis 205
paranoid schizophrenia 206
parasuicide 275
paroxetine 75
personality disorders 153–163
   borderline personality disorder
      155–157
   dependent personality disorder
      162
   dissociative identity disorder
      158–159

personality disorders—*contd.*
   multiple personality disorder
      158–159
   psychopathy 160–161, 162–163
phobias
   agoraphobia 13–15
   cat 31–33
   dog 150
post-natal depression 78, 93, 94–95,
   96–97
   accepting treatment 95
   antidepressants and breastfeeding
      96
   avoiding antidepressants 97
   prevention 94–95, 96–97
   subsequent pregnancies 94
   support 94
post-traumatic stress disorder 129,
   144, 232
premenstrual syndrome (PMS)
   187–188
   keeping a mood diary 187
   symptoms 187
   treatment 188
professional patient syndrome
   225
psychiatric disorders
   dealing with people recovering
      from 148–149
   respecting patient 149
   stigma 148
   violence and 148
psychiatric hospital, compulsory
   admission to 123–124,
   246–247
psychiatric illnesses
   bio-psycho-social elements
      150
   feigning 129–130
   medication and other treatment
      150–151
   repeat admissions to psychiatric
      hospitals 150–151
   treating causes 151
psychiatric services 165–175
   confidentiality of doctors 174–175
   disadvantages 172

psychiatric services—*contd.*
  options 170–171
  organisation 172–173
  private treatment 171, 173
psychiatrists 167–169
  analysis 167
  consultations 167–168
  private treatment 171, 173
psycho-education, bipolar depression 78, 81
psychoanalysis 167, 179, 180
psychological damages, pursuing case for 119–120
psychological debriefing 38–39
psychological therapies 177–184
  cognitive therapy 182–184
  jargon 179–181
  schizophrenia and 214–215
psychopathic personality disorder 162–163
psychopathy
  features 160
  inheritance of 160–161
  treatment 161
psychosexual disorders 185–201
  homosexuality 191–192
  impotence 193–194
  menopause 189–190
  painful sexual intercourse 195–197
  premenstrual syndrome (PMS) 187–188
  sexual abuse 198–199, 200–201
psychotherapy 156, 214

rapid cycling bipolar disorder 80, 82
recurrent depressive disorder 78
religious mania 141–142
repression 180
Ritalin 138
ruminations 24, 26

schizophrenia 129, 203–220
  amphetamines and 260
  biological changes in the brain 210
  counselling 214, 217, 219
  family relationships and 211–213

schizophrenia—*contd.*
  "hebephrenic" 129
  inheritance of 209–210
  medication 150, 214–215, 216, 217, 219
  necessity of medication 219
  omega-3 oil treatment 4
  overcoming the stigma 219–220
  paranoia 205–206
  positive and negative symptoms 216
  psychotherapy 214
  relapse 211, 212, 219
  split personality 207, 208
  suicide rates 211
  support from friends and family 220
  talking treatment 214
  theories 211
  tranquillizer treatment 216–218
  triggers 209–210, 260
  violent behaviour and 208, 219–220
Schizophrenia Ireland 217
seasonal affective disorder (SAD) 78, 98–99
  features of 98
  light therapy 98–99
  occurrence 98
  self-help 99
self-harm 142, 148, 155, 156, 182, 269, 275, 276
Seroxat 75–76
sexual abuse 198–199, 200–201
  clinical depression due to 198
  medication 200
  supportive parents 198
  therapists 200
  therapy 198–199, 201
sexual intercourse, painful 195–196
shoplifting 127–128
  forgetfulness and 127
  informing your family 127
  kleptomania and 128
shyness 28–30, 182
social anxiety (social phobia) 28–30
  negative effects 28

Index

social anxiety (social phobia)—*contd.*
   panic and fear 28
   techniques to cope with 29
   therapy 29
sodium valproate 83
somatoform disorders 221–227
   malingering 223–224
   Munchausen's syndrome 225–227
split personality, schizophrenia and 207, 219–220
spontaneous depression 90
St John's Wort 3–4
   drug and food interactions 5–6
   effectiveness in treating depression 5
   safety and side effects 6
steroids, side effects 146–147
stress 18, 229–240
   antidepressants and 236–237
   avoiding stressors 238–239
   definition 231
   depression and 234–235
   features 232
   negative coping skills 232
   normal versus abnormal 231–232
   overwork 238–240
   positive coping skills 232
   reactions to 232
   self-help 237
   support from others 239
   symptom reduction 239
   symptom relief 237
   unhappiness and 234–235
substance abuse 241–263
   alcohol problems 243–252
   amphetamines 259–260
   cannabis 253–254
   cocaine 255–256
   ecstasy 257–258
   heroin 261–263
suicidal person
   contacting your doctor 270, 274
   help for 270
   talking and listening to 269
suicidal thoughts
   acknowledging problem 274
   causes 273

suicidal thoughts—*contd.*
   clinical depression and 268
   professional help 267–268, 272, 273, 276
   taking seriously 267
   talking over 269, 271
suicide 47–48, 53–55, 265–279
   attempted 275–276
   bereavement after 47–48, 53–55
   community response 278
   copy-cat suicide 277–279
   emotions of bereaved 53
   helping the bereaved 54
   media coverage 277–278
   parasuicide 275
superego 179–180

talking treatments 78, 80, 151, 177–184
   cognitive therapy 182–184
   jargon 179–181
   schizophrenia and 214–215
tranquillizers 16–17, 19, 36–37, 71
   benzodiazepine (minor) 16–17, 34–35, 37, 216
   dependence 34–35
   major tranquillizers 16, 216
   minor tranquillizers 16–17, 34–35, 37, 216
   prescriptions for 37
   withdrawal from 34–35

unconscious fears 179
unipolar disorder 92

vaginismus 195, 196
vascular dementia 59–60
Viagra 195

"Werther Effect" 277
wills, validity of 125–126
work, problems at 36–37, 238–229
worrying 18–19
   causes of excessive 18–19
   necessity for medication 19
   reducing anxiety 19